I0428706

100 Push-ups

The Ultimate System for Consistent Push-up Progress

By: Eric Bowles

Copyright © 2011 Eric R. Bowles

All rights reserved. No part of this book, text, photographs or illustrations may be reproduced or transmitted in any form or by means by print, photoprint, microfilm, microfiche, photocopier, internet or in any way known or as yet unknown, or stored in a retrieval system, without written permission obtained beforehand by the author.

ISBN-10: 1470009382
ISBN-13: 978-1470009380

DISCLAIMER

The techniques, ideas, and suggestions in this document are not intended as a substitute for proper medical advice. Always consult a qualified health care provider before performing any new exercise or exercise technique, particularly if you are pregnant, nursing, elderly, or if you have any chronic or recurring conditions. Any application of the techniques, ideas, and suggestions in this document is at the reader's sole discretion and risk.

The author of this document makes no warranty of any kind in regard to the content of this document, including, but not limited to, any implied warranties of merchantability or fitness for any particular purpose. The author of this document is not liable or responsible to any person or entity for any errors contained in this document, or for any incidental, or consequential damage, or any injury of any kind caused or alleged to be caused directly or indirectly by the information contained within.

CONTENTS

WHY YOU ARE READING THIS BOOK

I will assume that if you're reading this book you have at least some interest in increasing the number of pushups you can do. Maybe you've been trying to increase your pushups for a long time, maybe it's a recent obsession or maybe you just have the slightest inkling of interest and curiosity to see if it's possible. Maybe you're just looking to become more physically fit or find a workout you can do at home. Whatever your motivation I hope this book will give you what you are looking for. If you don't have any interest in increasing your pushups then this is an odd choice of book for you however I hope that what's contained in it will inspire you and light a desire in you to increase the number of pushups you can do too.

Whatever your reason is, I've written this book to help you achieve your goal by using a simple, efficient system that will help you gradually increase the number of pushups you can do. Keep in mind that even though the system is simple and won't require a lot of time, it will require effort and a little bit of mental toughness; I want you to understand this from the get go. Your success using this program is completely up to you. I can give you the system, the advice, and all the tips and tricks in the world but unless you apply them with consistency and determination nothing will come of it.

Personally I hope you make a commitment to take action and then follow through; becoming better at anything takes effort but the rewards are worth it. In the case of pushups there aren't many people who can do 100 pushups in a row without stopping, there aren't very many that can even do fifty for that matter. It's interesting how just being able to do something like pushups (which seem so insignificant to most of everyday life) better than most people can actually increase your confidence. And although it doesn't happen often, occasionally I've found myself in the middle of impromptu pushup contests and personally, I want to be able to perform well at these rather than shy away from the challenge.

Before I get into the meat of this book I want you to understand a little bit about me and what prompted me to write it. So please sit back and get comfortable, I hope to educate, entertain, and give you a system you can use for the rest of your life. Enjoy.

INTRODUCTION TO MY STORY

Fitness is an important part of my life and has been for a long time. I was overweight as a child. I still remember how uncomfortable I felt at school being one of the biggest kids in the class. I never felt comfortable in my clothes, I wished they would hide the fact that I was fat rather than accentuate it. Fortunately I was good natured so most people liked me, but there were of course those who made fun of me because of my size. I certainly understand what it's like to be overweight, uncomfortable, and to wish you were invisible. If you've never experienced that I'm happy for you, if you have, I feel for you.

That being said, I want you to understand that I truly believe the past does not dictate the future. We shape the future based on our decisions now. Your present situation and abilities have no bearing on the future unless you continue to make the decisions that have gotten you where you are. If you want to be different in the future you have to change the decisions you make today, I am proof of that; but enough philosophy.

When I got into middle school I decided to try out for sports. I played football and wrestled that year and while I didn't excel at either, the practices and training I did sparked something inside me that has grown to be one of the most important things in my life, a love for fitness. I realized I didn't have to be the fat kid anymore, I began to study and apply everything I could to try to become healthy and strong. I wanted to be a good athlete but more than that I wanted to have and maintain optimal health for the rest of my life. A funny thing happened over the course of middle school and high school as a result of this. I grew about a foot and a half taller but graduated high school at the same weight I entered middle school. I've always found that amusing.

After high school I could have easily stopped working out. There weren't any more sports to train for and all my other friends stopped working out, but fitness had become a part of who I was, and I was fueled by memories of being overweight and a promise to myself to never let my body become like that again. Living in a very small town and having limited access to a gym meant I often had to improvise to work out, but I always found a way and always made the time.

The program I'm going to share with you was developed by me at a time in my life when I basically had no access to any type of gym or training facility of any kind. I was living in the Ukraine at the time, and while it was a very enjoyable time in my life, I was only ever able to go to a gym a couple times in the whole two years I was there.

Knowing that I was going to the Ukraine for a long period of time and the challenges of staying in shape while far from home and without a gym, I decided to set a goal to help keep me on track and give me a reason to continue training. The goal was something I had never done before but thought it would be fun to achieve. I had total confidence that if I applied myself consistently I would be able to do it. My goal was to be able to do 200 pushups in a row, without stopping, by the time I came back to the states. That may seem like a crazy goal to some but I was bound and determined to do it, and even though I got off to a slow start, I eventually developed a system so elegant and effective that I believe anybody can use it to achieve any pushup goal they desire. This program will work for both men and women but before I continue with the rest of this story and the program let's go over a few fundamental things about the pushup so that we're all on the same page.

FIRST THINGS FIRST, WHAT IS A PUSHUP?

I would hope that everyone knows what a pushup is but just to be sure, here is a brief description of a basic pushup.

A pushup is typically a body weight exercise. The exerciser places their hands on the floor a little wider than shoulder width apart, elbows pointing back and away from the body at about 45 degrees, arms fully extended. The body is rigid through the spine, hips and legs as the feet are extended back as far as they can go; the toes and balls of the feet are placed on the floor. The point where the feet touch the floor is the point about which the body rotates while the exerciser bends at the elbow and shoulder to lower the chest to the floor. Once the arm reaches at least a 90 degree bend at the elbow the person can then push on the floor through the hands to straighten the arm and return to the starting position.

There are many variations to the pushup which can make performing the exercise easier or more difficult; those will be covered later, for now what's described above will be our model pushup.

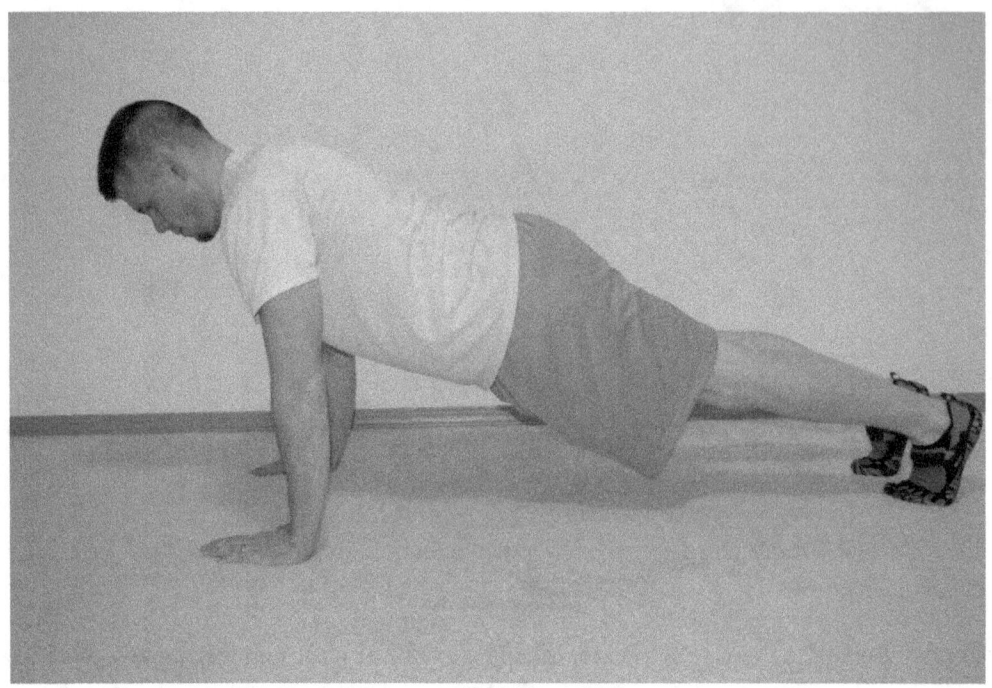

Figure. 1. Basic pushup start/finish position

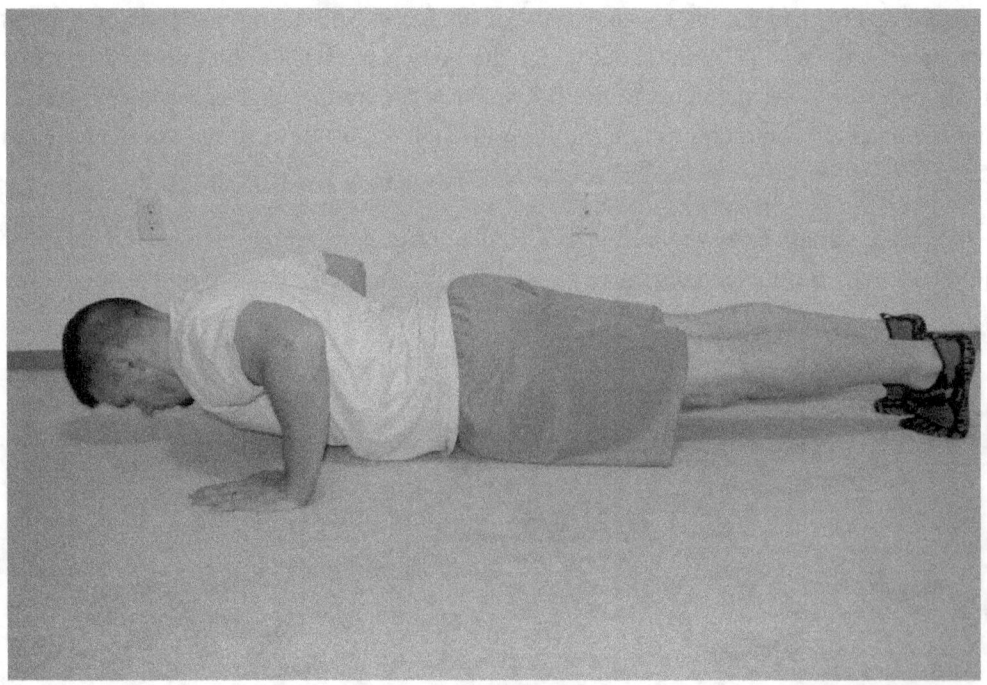

Figure. 2. Basic pushup lowered position

WHY DO PUSHUPS?

Everyone should do pushups on a regular basis; it's a great exercise for many reasons. One reason is that anybody can do them. That being said, if you've never done one before or if you're extremely out of shape you may not be able to do one this instant but you can work into it. With the right training and progression anyone can get to the point where they can do pushups.

The pushup is also a great exercise because there is no equipment required. The pushup is a body weight exercise, so as long as you have a body (which I'm assuming you do), and a few square feet to work in (which is easy enough to find), you can get a good workout based solely on pushups. That's not to say that you can't use various pieces of equipment to increase or decrease the difficulty or add variety, but it certainly isn't necessary. The fact that the pushup is a body weight exercise gives it some other advantages too. For instance, there are some distinct neurological benefits that come from moving your body through space, our bodies are made to move through space and because of this, adaptation occurs quickly.

An interesting thing about pushups is that a lot of them can be done without putting an extreme amount of stress on the body. This gives the pushup some advantages over other exercises, for one, it means you can practice a lot. You can do multiple pushup workouts each week, this gives you the ability to improve relatively quickly. I am all for lifting heavy weights to gain strength; I've lifted weights consistently for over fifteen years. When lifting weights, if you want to continue to make progress over time, you have to take scheduled breaks to let your body recover from the intense training. But using body weight exercises like pushups and body weight squats, you can work out and make progress for a much longer period of time before you reach that point where the intensity is so high you must take longer, more frequent breaks. This means you can continue to improve for extended periods of time.

The pushup can build muscle, strength and endurance. This is important because the more muscle you have and the stronger you are the easier it will be to age. We all age, it's unavoidable, personally I want to be strong and active well into old age and it's absolutely possible to do with a good training program.

On a side note, in a world that values bodies that look good, the emphasis always seems to be on losing weight. When people say this what they're really saying is "I want my body to look better." Unfortunately most people don't understand that for a body to look better it's not about "losing weight" it's about eliminating excess body fat (not dietary fat, that is completely different), and gaining or maintaining muscle mass. Our muscles are what give our bodies the nice shape we are after, the fat gives our bodies the shape we don't want and in all honesty it doesn't matter what either of these substances weighs, that's just the pull of gravity on the different cells. No one should care about the gravitational pull on cells. What matters is how many of each kind of cell is in your body. If muscle weighed 100 times what fat weighed and you lost 100 units of fat and gained one unit of muscle you would still weigh the same amount but would look a whole lot better. The moral of the side note is that building muscle is a good thing. Not only will it make you stronger, it will also burn more calories each day than an equal amount of fat.

One of my favorite reasons and maybe one of the best reasons the pushup is a great exercise is that, despite the simple up and down motion, the pushup is a full body exercise. Maintaining the pushup position activates to some degree almost all the major muscle groups in the body, thus strengthening nearly the whole body at the same time. Not only are all the muscles strengthened, they're strengthened in a way that's very functional. Muscles are made to work together in groups; it's very rare that you only use one muscle during a task. Just think about walking, your leg muscles, your butt muscles, the stabilizers in your back and abdomen, your shoulders and neck, all work together to help your body walk without falling over. Picking something up off the ground employs the same principle, multiple groups of muscles working together to accomplish a task. The pushup helps train almost all your muscles at once while teaching them to work together to perform a task, that's pretty awesome. To illustrate this better we'll now go over the muscles that are trained while doing pushups.

THE PUSHUP MUSCLES

As mentioned before, the pushup activates almost every major muscle group in the body. Let's go over those now, starting with the most obvious ones.

The **Pectoralis** major and minor, better known as the "pecs", are the large muscles across the upper chest. These attach your breastbone to the humerus (the bone of the upper arm) and contract to bring the humerus forward and down.

The **Deltoids**, especially the front and mid (top) deltoids, are the shoulder muscles. They attach to the collar bone and the humerus and contract to bring the arm forward and up.

The **Triceps** are the major muscles on the back of the upper arm. They attach at the top of the humerus and down at the forearm around the elbow. When they contract they straighten the arm at the elbow.

These three muscle groups work together anytime you push something away from your body. If you were lying on a bench and pushing a weight up these would be the muscles you would be working. A few of the muscles in your back would activate to stabilize you a bit but the bench would do most of the stabilization. However, when you're in the pushup position you can't rely on anything to stabilize you except yourself. Your body has to activate lots of different muscles to maintain its rigidity as gravity tries to pull you down.

The secondary muscles the body uses to maintain stability and rigidity are for the most part used isometrically which means they're being flexed but not causing movement. There are nine groups of muscles used this way, each is described below.

The first two sets of secondary muscles are used to maintain the position of the scapula. The first of these are the **rhomboids.** These are short muscles in the upper back that connect the spine to the inner scapula. The second set of muscles responsible for scapula stability are the **serratus** muscles located on the side of the body under the upper arm, they wrap around to the back and attach to the outside of the scapula. During a pushup these muscles hold the scapula in place so it doesn't slide across to the center of the back and cause the chest to sag down. If your chest sags down when your arms are locked out straight it's because your rhomboids and serratus muscles are not holding the scapula in place.

The next two sets of secondary muscles are used for shoulder stability. The **rotator cuff** is a group of muscles that run from the scapula to the top of the humerus; their job is to keep the humerus locked into the shoulder joint so that the deltoids can move the humerus more efficiently. Weakness in these muscles would cause the humerus to slide out of the joint and decrease the efficiency of the deltoids. Next, the **posterior deltoid** is the part of the deltoid that attaches the humerus to the scapula. During the pushup it also serves to stabilize the humerus in the shoulder joint.

The next three muscle groups work together to maintain the stability of the abdomen and are the first link in the rigidity that must be maintained between the upper and lower body. These three muscle groups are the **rectus abdominus** (otherwise known as the "abs"), the **transverse abdominus**, which are on each side of the abs and connect to the rib cage, hips and fascia of the lower back (or lumbar spine) and act as a belt when flexed, and the **erector spinae** which are the long muscles on each side of the spine which run from the pelvis up to the middle of the back. When these three muscle groups are flexed together it keeps the lower back rigid so the stomach can't sag towards the floor.

The last major muscle groups that are activated during pushups are in the legs. The **gluteals,** or butt muscles, connect the pelvis to the top of the femur (upper leg bone). When the gluteus maximus is flexed it brings the femur in line with the upper body. If you feel that your hips are starting to sag as you do pushups, one of the best things to do is focus on flexing your butt, it will help pull your body back into alignment. The second major muscle group in the leg that is activated while doing pushups is the **quadriceps**. These are the four large muscles in the front of the leg; their major function is to straighten the leg at the knee. These muscles must be activated while in pushup position to maintain straight legs. The three muscles of the lower leg, commonly called the **calf** muscles, are also activated to some degree to maintain the rigidity of the ankle. It is possible to do pushups without activating these muscles but it's easier to maintain good form if you keep the ankle rigid.

As you can see, the pushup is an amazing exercise for stimulating nearly all the muscles in your body at the same time. Just a quick count shows that twelve major muscle groups are at work if you don't count the deltoids twice. You'd be hard-pressed to find another exercise as simple as the pushup that activates so many muscles at the same time.

Of the major muscle groups in the body, five are not stimulated much while doing pushups, these include: the latissimus dorsi and trapezius which are the large muscles of the mid and upper back, the hamstrings which are located on the back of the upper legs, and the biceps and forearm muscles of the arm.

It's important to maintain balanced strength around each joint of the body in order to maintain proper joint function and optimal health. This means we can't neglect to strengthen these muscles as we're increasing the strength of the pushup muscles, to do so would eventually lead to bad posture, joint pain, fat gain and possibly even injury. This program has been designed with a balanced approach in mind so that, while the focus and main goal will be to increase the number of pushups you can do, the end result will strengthen the whole body.

MY STORY CONTINUED

With the basics of pushups out of the way I want to continue my story about how I developed my program and tell you what my end results were.

When I first left home on my trip to the Ukraine I didn't really have a set plan in mind as to how I was going to achieve my goal, but I knew I needed to do two things at the very beginning to set some parameters so I could track my progress. The first thing I needed to do was find out how many pushups I could do without stopping at the beginning of my trip. The second thing I needed to do was determine my definition of stopping.

I realized that when doing pushups, even if I wasn't going up and down, my body was still doing work by maintaining its rigidity, but I also knew that if my primary movement muscles stopped moving for too long they would be able to recover a large enough amount of energy to be able to continue doing pushups as long as I could keep my body stiff. I decided that, when in the up position, if I had to take more than two breaths before doing another pushup then that was too long of a break and the set was over. That way I wasn't able to stay in the up position for five to ten seconds before doing another pushup, it made it so my slowest pace (which of course was towards the end of a set) was about two to three seconds per pushup. After two breaths I went down no matter what and if I couldn't come back up in good form the set was over.

So the very first week out I did a max set of sixty-two. That wasn't too bad but it certainly wasn't close to 200, I had a lot of work to do.

Initially I had no real system of training. I would do a few sets of pushups before I went to bed each day, sometimes every other day, and call it good; usually doing rep ranges around two thirds my current max. I made some progress doing this and got my max up to sixty-eight by the end of the month. I think most of that improvement was just my body getting used to doing more pushups.

At the end of the first month an unexpected twist came to me when I acquired a pair of pushup bars. If you don't know what a pushup bar is, let me explain. Pushup bars are a set of small handles on legs that elevate your upper body about five inches. They allow your chest to go lower than it could if doing pushups with your hands on the floor, this increases the difficulty of a pushup significantly (see Appendix A). I decided to give them a try and found my initial max on the pushup bars was thirty-two, over fifty percent less than doing normal pushups! I was amazed at the degree of difficulty they added but enjoyed the new challenge.

I began doing all my workouts on my new pushup bars but my training plan was still pretty vague. In the mornings I would wake up and do an aerobic type workout for twenty to twenty-five minutes and then at night before going to bed I would do a few sets of pushups and then test my strength at the end of the week.

Doing this I was able to make progress even without a good plan, which is a testament to how well the body adapts to body weight exercises, but I was not making the kind of progress I needed to in order to get my pushups up to 200 without stopping by the time I went home.

Looking back on this time I have tried to pinpoint a specific event that led to the development of the program I eventually made but I've been unable to determine what it was. I think it just slowly morphed into a system that made sense to me and which started giving me fast, consistent results. I do know that it took about a year for it to fully develop into the program I used for the remainder of my trip, and the week that I first implemented the finished system my max on the pushup bars was forty-eight.

The first thing I realized while developing my system was that I didn't need to do pushups every day, I found that three days a week worked great. That gave my body time to rest and recover for at least one day between each workout. Convenient for my situation I scheduled my pushup training time like this: Monday, pushup training, Wednesday, pushup training, Saturday, pushup max. That schedule seemed to be the perfect balance between enough time doing pushups and enough time to recover.

I eventually realized I needed a way to indicate when it was time to increase the intensity of my regular pushup training days. Once that was implemented my training became very systematic, easy to track and make progress. I also implemented a penalty for not reaching training goals as an incentive to push myself, but also to help me get stronger faster if I was consistently missing my goals.

Once my system was in place my pushup ability quickly started to improve. It wasn't easy; I had to push myself each week. There were times when it was painful but I was having so much fun making progress I didn't care. My max test became one of the things I looked forward to all week.

On my non-pushup training days I eventually created systems to develop the other muscle groups and maintain balanced strength. Looking back on my non-pushup training systems and knowing what I know now I would have done things a bit differently, which I am doing in this training program (Aren't you lucky to be benefiting from my extra years of experience?), however, I was able to get to the point where I could do some pretty cool stuff. I could do two, five-minute wall-sits in a row with only a two-minute break in between, I could also do two three-minute hand stands with the same break. I had acquired a dumbbell as well as a chest expander with springs and could do all kinds of crazy amounts of reps with those things by the time I came home.

All that is well and good but I'm sure the thing you're most interested in is the number of pushups I was able to do by the time I came home. Did I reach my goal? Well yes and no. In all honesty, for some reason, I never did a max with regular pushups the week I came home (I still can't figure out why). But I did do a max with my pushup bars and I was able to do 109 reps before failure. I was pretty happy with that number because in my mind it was logical to think I could do about twice as many normal pushups as pushups on the bars. If you recall, when I started using the bars, my max went from sixty-eight to thirty-two, if you reverse that ratio 109 bar pushups would equate to 231 regular pushups. Even if that wouldn't have been the exact number, I was confident that I would be able to get close to 200, the limiting factor would probably have been maintaining a plank position long enough to finish, even at one rep per second that's well over three minutes.

In the years since then I've never found a system that gave me such great results as quickly and consistently. I've tried sharing my program with friends and family but none of them ever used it because they didn't really have an interest in doing lots of pushups. That is why I am sharing it here. I want you to be able to benefit from my system and since it's likely I've never met you, and will probably never have that privilege, this book is the most logical way to reach you. So without further ado, here is the training system I used to go from forty-eight bar pushups to 109 in a little under a year. I'm confident it will help increase the number of pushups you can do too.

THE PROGRAM

So let's get into the program. Before I lay it out you need to understand a couple things. First, this was my strength training at the time I was living in the Ukraine; I have never tested this with a concurrent strength training program with weights. Second, I did these workouts about an hour before bed; I also did twenty to twenty-five minutes of cardio-boxing type workouts each morning.

I want you to understand this because you may get different results if you do this workout along with heavy weight training or if you do it right after an intense cardio workout, I was fresh when I did these workouts. It's intended to be a strength training workout that can be completed in fifteen minutes or less. That being said, because it's mainly a body weight workout you may be able to incorporate it into a weight training workout and still see results, that's something you'd have to test yourself.

The workout is a seven-day training plan, obviously that fits easily into a week. The protocol is laid out like this:

Day 1: Pushup focus

Day 2: Auxiliary and muscle balancing

Day 3: Pushup focus

Day 4: Auxiliary and muscle balancing

Day 5: Auxiliary and muscle balancing

Day 6: Pushup focus

Day 7: Rest

What follows is the workout for each day. I'm going to lay it out the way I developed and used it. I will also give you some advice for tweaks or adjustments that can be made to suit your individual needs/circumstances.

DAY 1: PUSHUP FOCUS

1A. **Pushups:** 3 Sets

Rules:

1: Each set of pushups should have five more reps than the previous set. Example: set 1 has 20 pushups, set 2 has 25 pushups, and set 3 has 30 pushups.

2: On the last set do as many reps as you can (max), keeping in mind that you should not rest more than two breaths between any repetition and that the minimum (goal) number of pushups is ten more than your first set.

3: Penalty pushups: If on any set you fail to reach your goal number of pushups, take a twenty to thirty-second break, and then do twice the number of pushups you missed your goal by. Example: set 3 goal = 30 pushups, achieved 27 pushups, difference = 30 − 27 = 3, 2 x difference = 2 x 3 = 6 pushups. Do six pushups after twenty to thirty seconds of rest.

4: If you do not achieve all your penalty pushups, wait another thirty to forty seconds and do the difference of the penalty pushups missed. Example: 6 penalty pushups, 4 accomplished, 6 − 4 = 2, 2 x 2 = 4 more penalty pushups.

5: If you do not achieve the second set of penalty pushups, move on.

6: Advancing: Once you can do ten to fifteen more pushups than required on the last set, increase the starting number of pushups by five and use that as your new starting set. Example: Initial set is 20 reps, final set requires 30 reps. Performed 42 reps on the final set, 12 more than required, on the next workout start with 25 reps for the first set. New set goals are 25, 30, and 35 reps.

1B. **Abdominal exercises:** 2-3 Sets

Perform a set of abdominal exercises immediately after each set of pushups (unless you are waiting to do penalty pushups). After the abdominal exercise, rest anywhere between thirty seconds to one minute before doing the next set of pushups. The exercises I recommend are as follows:

Planks: Start at thirty seconds and work up to two minutes, if you can do two minutes, include stability ball planks and/or single-leg planks.

Side Planks: Start at thirty seconds and work up to two minutes. If you can do a two-minute side plank, put your elbow on a stability disk or stability ball.

Ab-wheel rollout: Start with a low number (these can be challenging), eventually try to work up to being able to do as many as your age (of course this exercise requires an ab-wheel).

Leg raises: Lie with your back to the floor and lift your legs from the floor until they're perpendicular to the ceiling (if you have the equipment, hanging leg raises are even better). If you can't do this exercise with your legs straight, bend your knees enough to allow you to do at least ten reps. When you can do thirty reps with your legs bent, begin doing reps with your legs straighter until you can do reps with your legs fully extended.

Avoid crunches and sit-ups. They really aren't that effective for building a strong abdomen. The abdominals are stability muscles and receive the most benefit from training when they are trained as such. They are not meant to flex your lower spine over and over. This can actually put your back at risk of injury. The only crunch I recommend is a stretch-crunch where you lay back over a stability ball stretching your abs so that your upper body is situated below horizontal and then flex your abs to bring your torso just above horizontal. This gives your abs a good stretch and decent workload without extreme forward flexion of the spine.

DAY 2: AUXILIARY AND MUSCLE BALANCING

1A. Lunges/Step-ups: 4 Sets

These exercises can be performed isometrically or as a regular repetition movement. Two sets should be performed per leg (left set, right set, left set, right set).

Rules/insight:

Lunges: Step with only one leg at a time until the set is done, do not alternate legs during the set. Start with ten reps per leg. The second set for each leg should have at least five more reps per leg, when ten more reps per leg is possible on the second set, make that the new starting point. Do not go over thirty reps per leg per set. If you get to this point start adding weights, do side lunges or step-ups.

Lunge variations: If you step forward to lunge, most of the training will be in the quads or the front of the leg, if you step back (reverse lunge), most of the training will be in the hamstrings and butt. The reverse lunge is highly recommended as the pushups will give your quads at least some isometric training. Side lunges are also possible and will add a degree of difficulty if regular and reverse lunges become too easy.

Isometric holds: These must be done with 90 degree angles maintained at the knees and hips. Start with thirty-second to one-minute holds per leg. The second set must be at least fifteen to thirty seconds longer than the first. Once the second set can be held for one minute longer than the first, increase the time of the first set by thirty seconds on the next workout.

Step-ups: If lunges become too easy you can switch to step-ups, they work many of the same muscles as a reverse lunge but are more difficult. Progress with step-ups the same way you progress with lunges. Don't do more than thirty reps per leg, per set; add weight if you need to.

1B. Body weight Rows/Pull-ups: 3 Sets

Preform one set of body weight rows or pull-ups between each set of lunges or step-ups. These exercises can be performed isometrically or as a regular repetition movement.

Rules/Insight:

Use the same rules of progression as you use for pushups (see Day 1), the only difference being the number of reps you add per set. If doing body weight rows, five to ten reps per set will be good, if doing pull-ups, anywhere between one and three is typically adequate. Also, if doing pull-ups, when you can do five more than your final goal set, increase the starting set by one or two on the next workout.

If you don't have a bar to do body weight rows or pull-ups you can use a sturdy table, or a partner who is willing to hold your hands

When doing body weight rows, the closer your feet are to your butt the easier they will be, the farther out your feet are the harder they will be.

Row up till your chest touches or nearly touches the bar; pull-up till your chin is above the bar.

Isometric Rows/Pull-ups: Use the same rules for isometric rows and pull-ups as outlined previously for lunges. Elbows should be bent 90 degrees for all holds. Try to increase the time you can hold the position in perfect form.

DAY 3: PUSHUP FOCUS

Repeat the workout as outlined in Day 1, adjust starting reps if needed.

1A. Pushups: 3 Sets

1B. Abdominal exercises: 2-3 Sets

DAY 4: AUXILIARY AND MUSCLE BALANCING

1A. Handstands: 2 Sets

Rules/Insight:

These are handstands done against a wall as an isometric exercise with arms straight.

Start with thirty-second to one-minute holds. The second set must be at least fifteen to thirty seconds longer than the first. If you can hold the second set for a minute longer than the first set, increase the time you hold the first set by thirty seconds in the next workout.

If you can't do a handstand, start by holding something above your head. Once you reach the point where you can hold it above your head for five minutes, switch to a heavier object or attempt to do a handstand. Handstands can be challenging, start slow with this one, you don't want to fall on your head.

When you're in handstand position, tuck your chin to your chest, do not tilt your head back and look at the floor, if you do you can potentially break many small blood vessels and have hundreds of little red spots all across your face.

If you can handstand for at least five minutes or want to increase the difficulty, bend your elbows.

1B. Wall-sit: 1-2 Sets

Rules/Insight:

This is an isometric exercise.

Place your back against a wall, feet out in front of you about shoulder width apart, knees bent at 90 degrees.

Hold that position at least as long as you hold your second isometric lunge from Day 2. If you don't perform isometric lunges on Day 2, try to start out with about thirty seconds to one minute. Try to increase your time each week.

If you would like, perform a second wall-sit after the second set of handstands. Follow the rules of progression in the second set as outlined for isometric lunges (see Day 2).

DAY 5: AUXILIARY AND MUSCLE BALANCING

Repeat the workout as outlined in Day 2, adjust starting reps if needed.

1A. Lunges/Step-ups: 4 Sets

1B. Body weight Rows/Pull-ups: 3 Sets

DAY 6: PUSHUP FOCUS

Max Day

Follow the protocol below:

1: Do five to ten pushups to warm up. Do these at a normal pace just to get a bit of blood flowing to the muscles and to prep your muscles for the max attempt. This should be a very minimal and very easy set so do what's easy for you. Wait about a minute before going on to the next set; keep your arms moving while you wait.

2: Maximum reps. Do pushups until failure. Failure occurs when you can no longer push your body up from the bottom position with good form. The longest allowable break between reps is two breaths (two to three seconds), a break longer than that also indicates the set's completion.

3: Rest for about thirty seconds to one minute and then do some very light abdominal work. (I recommend leg raises here as you have just finished a pretty intense plank, keep the reps low.) Rest for another thirty seconds to one minute before going on to step 4.

4: Maximum reps. Do a second set of pushups to failure. Use the reps of the first set as the goal for the second, however, if you don't reach that number there are no penalty pushups.

DAY 7: REST AND RECOVERY

SUMMING IT UP

So there you have it, the simple workout plan you can do at home to help you reach the capacity to be able to do 100 pushups in a row. As you can see, the system is short, simple, and because it mainly relies on body weight exercises, it can be repeated week after week for a long time. That being said, it may not be appropriate for you at your current level the way it's written so here are some things to consider before you implement it.

Be mindful about warming up your muscles before starting any exercise program. Some light stretching and dynamic movement before proceeding with the exercises will help lubricate the joints, warm up the muscles and prepare them for the work they're about to do. I didn't include any warm-ups or stretches in this program but I certainly recommend you do them. This becomes more important as you get older but even if you're young you should warm up, it's a good habit to get into and will save your body a lot of wear and tear as you age. Don't stretch too deep or hard before the workout, just light stretching and movement will be fine, a deeper stretch can be done after the workout is completed.

I've stated that you need to increase the number of pushups per set by five. This may not be appropriate for everyone, if you can't do twenty pushups yet it may be more appropriate to increase the reps by two each set, however if you can already do a lot of pushups a larger increase like seven to ten per set may be more beneficial. The five pushups per set increase I did was using pushup bars. If I had been doing regular pushups I may have used larger increases between sets. The amount of the step up is important and it needs to fit your ability. If you like the idea of adding five pushups per set, one way to implement it is to do pushups at a difficulty that will allow you to increase by five per set whether it's by using wall pushups, kneeling pushups, regular pushups or pushups on bars. Find the step up that works for you.

If you can't do a pushup yet you'll need to start with an exercise that's easier. Wall pushups are the easiest pushup exercise and progressions get harder from there. A wall pushup is performed by placing your arms out in front of you against a wall, as if doing a pushup on the ground, and placing your feet back so you are leaning against the wall. You then perform the same pushup movement as you would on the ground except your body is moving towards the wall. The closer your body gets to horizontal the more difficult the pushup will get, so when wall pushups get too easy (when you can do fifty to 100 reps per set) you can progress by leaning on a sturdy table or countertop, anything that will situate your body more horizontally. Eventually you will be able to do kneeling pushups, and then full pushups.

If you're doing kneeling pushups, understand that there will be a point where you'll need to graduate to full pushups. I recommend doing planks with your arms fully extended, as if in pushup position, between each set of kneeling pushups. Doing planks with arms fully extended between sets will condition the abs and prepare all your stabilization muscles for the full strain of regular pushups. You should also set a goal to transfer into doing regular pushups when you get to the point where you can do fifty or more reps per set on your knees.

I'm sure you've noticed there are a lot of maximal effort sets in this system. I realize these sets are difficult and can even be painful. This is why I stated at the beginning that it would require a bit of mental toughness. Don't be afraid of the pain (unless it's from an injury, then you should stop and seek professional advice and treatment). I can't give you the drive to push through the pain, that's something you have to find within yourself, but I know that if you can find that drive and apply it, great things will happen and you will achieve your goals. Once you reach your goal you will look back on the journey and see that pushing yourself was well worth it. Usually all it takes is enough mental toughness to do one more pushup than last time, if you can find that within yourself you will always make progress.

I tried to develop this system so that no equipment would be required. That being said, it may be helpful to have a dumbbell or two to increase the resistance for some of the exercises. The lunges and step-ups especially will benefit from the added resistance. The largest muscles in the body are in the legs and they can handle a lot of intensity. Holding a dumbbell or two while doing lunges, step-ups or isometric lunges will benefit your body immensely, plus, dumbbells can be used as pushup bars if you don't already have a set. Also, if you don't have a pull-up bar or a good table to do body weight rows, you can use the dumbbells to do dumbbell rows in conjunction with your lunges. Whether you do pull-ups, body weight rows or dumbbell rows it's important to not neglect exercising the back, especially when doing the amount of pushups this program requires. If you neglect your back your body will become unbalanced which can lead to pain or even injury.

Last of all I just want to mention that recovery is very important. The workout is not what makes you stronger, it's the recovery after the workout where your body improves itself. When you finish a workout you have to give your body the time and materials it needs to adapt. This means you need to eat good food and drink plenty of water each day. Most likely you will need to increase your protein consumption (most people don't eat enough protein) as well as your consumption of vegetables. Reduce the amount of processed foods you eat, especially refined sugars and flour products, our bodies were never made to digest these and they cause all sorts of problems which is beyond the scope of this book to describe. A good rule to follow is, if your great grandparents wouldn't know what it is, don't eat it. Finally, make sure you get enough sleep; this is when the majority of recovery and repair takes place. If you don't sleep enough it will take a long time to recover. I realize that our lives are such that getting enough sleep each night can be difficult but you must make it a priority if you want to see progress. If you find you're not making progress with the seven day cycle you may want to try and add another rest day or two somewhere in the program.

I wish you the best as you embark on your journey. I hope my insight, experience and system will be of use to you in your endeavor.

Good Luck!

Appendix A: Pushup Progression

Pushup progression: Below is a simple pushup progression from easy to difficult.

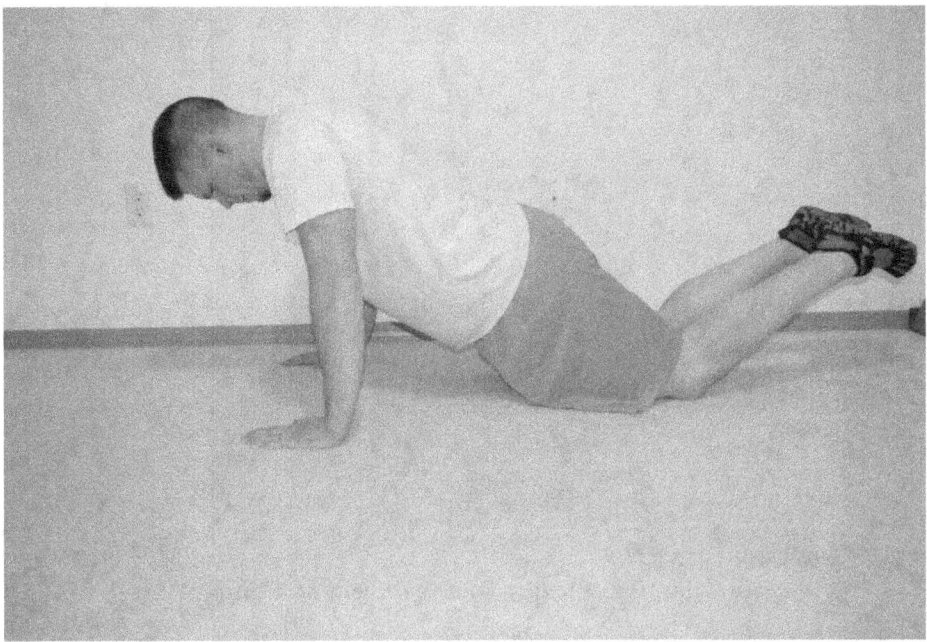

A1. Kneeling or sissy pushup

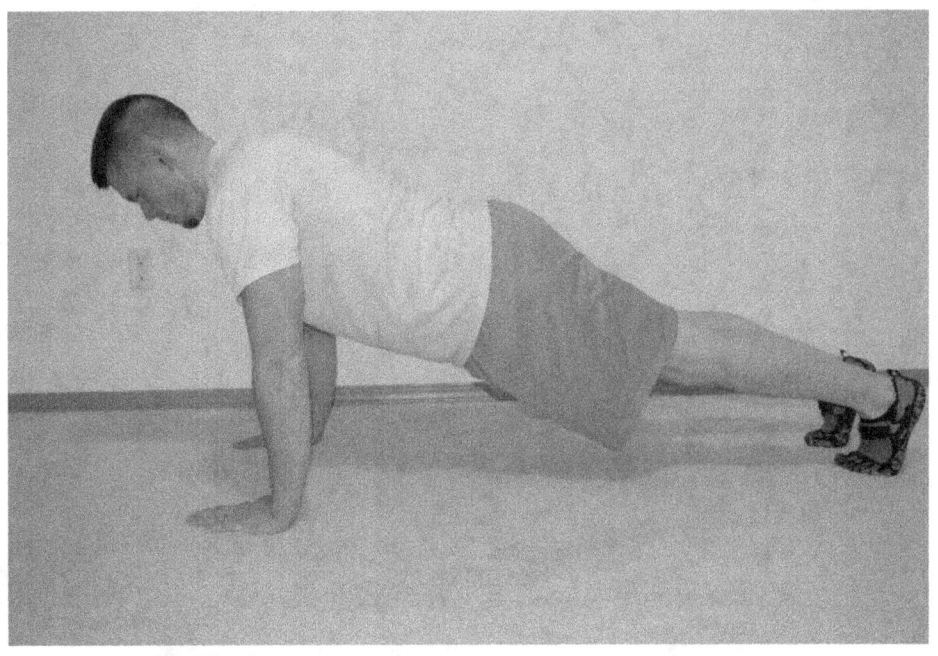

A2. Pushup

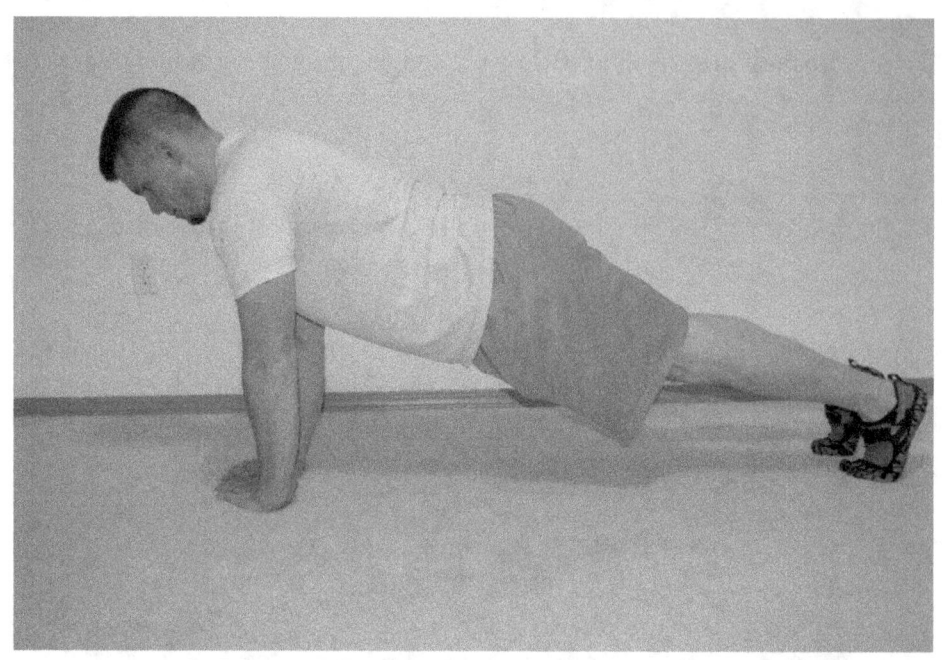

A3. Diamond Pushup (index fingers and thumbs touching)

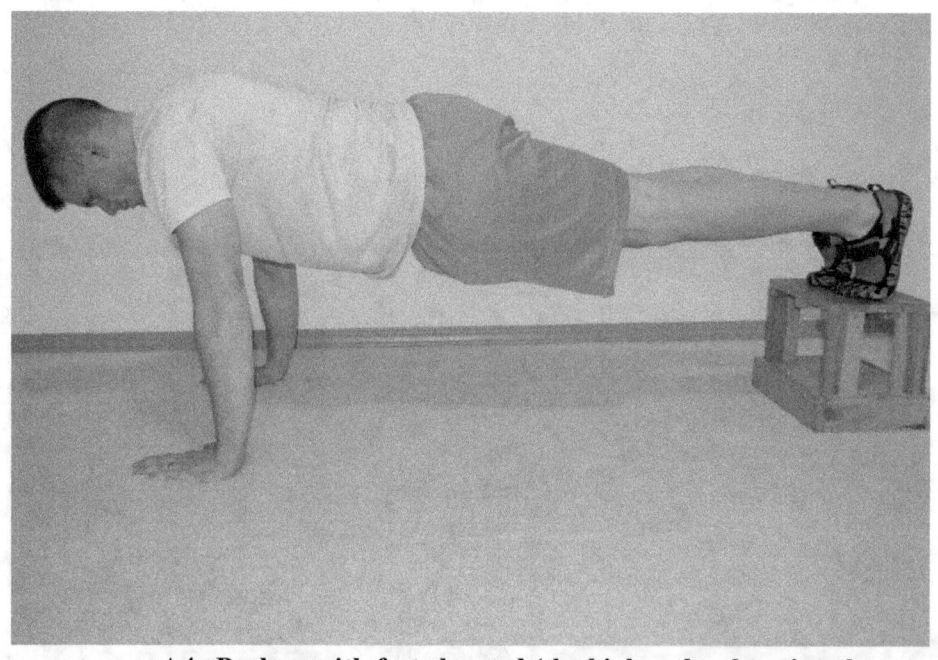

A4. Pushup with feet elevated (the higher the elevation the more difficult it gets)

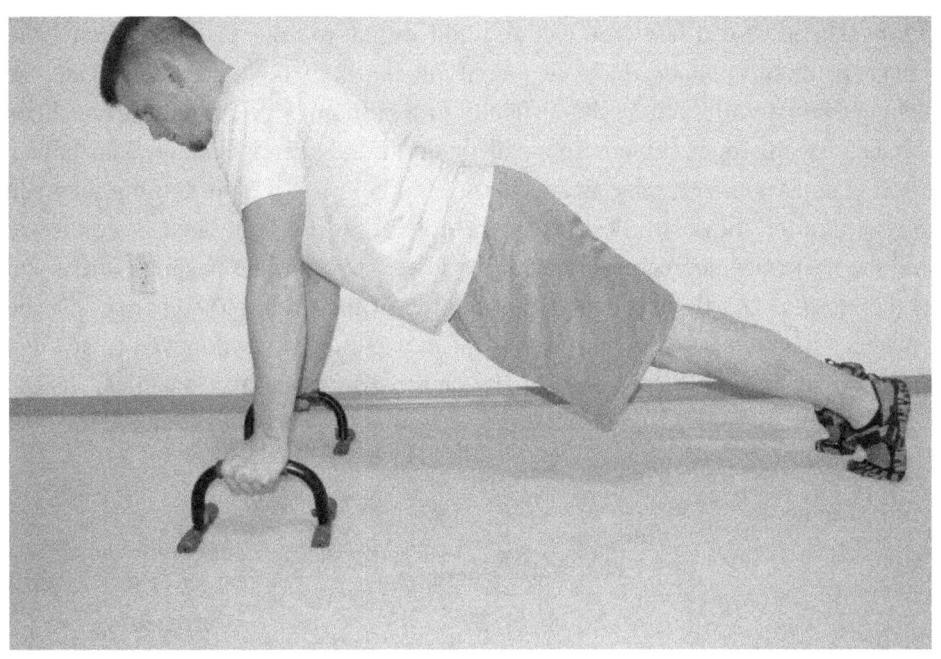

A5. Pushups on pushup bars

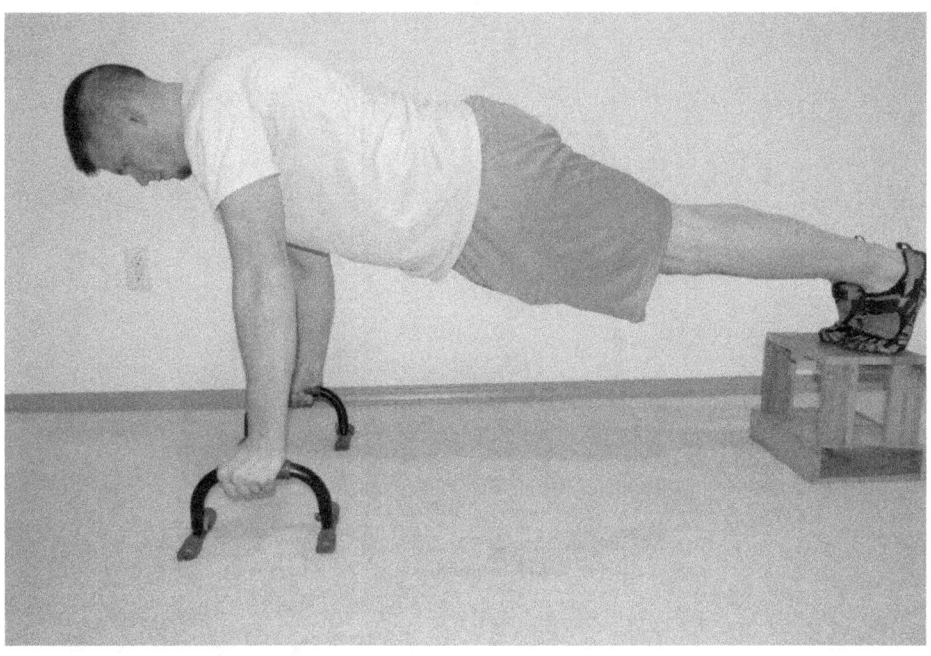

A6. Pushups on pushup bars, feet elevated

Beyond the progression shown here you can also add weight to your body to increase the difficulty. A weight vest, chains, bands, kids etc. anything that can be used to increase the resistance you're pushing against will increase the difficulty of a pushup. I've done lots of pushups with my kids on my back, not only does it increase the difficulty of the exercise but the kids have a good time too. Weight vests are okay as long as they're not too bulky, if they're too big they can really reduce the range of motion. Bands and chains can be good tools to use because as you lower yourself to the ground the resistance decreases so that at the lowest point of the pushup (where you will be the weakest) the resistance is the smallest and at the top of the pushup (where you will be the strongest) the resistance is greatest. You may also want to experiment with uneven (place one hand higher than the other by resting it on a few books or a ball) or one arm pushups. These variations will also increase the difficulty, and without the need of any specialized equipment.

Appendix B: Arm Orientation

The angle of your arm will determine which primary muscles will be doing the majority of the work as you do pushups. When I say "angle of the arm" I'm talking about the angle between your upper arm and your torso. There are three typical positions to discuss.

The first position is the most common and that is to have your arms out at a 45 degree angle. This position is what I would consider a regular pushup position. This position distributes the stress more or less equally between the triceps, pecs and deltoids and is a very natural position to be in. If you place your hands a little wider than shoulder width apart with your fingers pointed forward in line with your body, this should be the most natural and comfortable position to lower your body into.

The second position is to bring your upper arms and elbows to the side of your body as you descend. This position places a much higher load on the front deltoid and triceps muscles. To descend in this position you must place your hands directly under your shoulders, fingers pointed forward in line with your body. With arms extended you must rotate your arms slightly at the wrists and shoulders so your elbows are pointing towards your feet. As you descend it will feel as if your chest is moving forward slightly. This pushup position is a little more difficult than the regular 45 degree position described above.

The third position is to point your upper arms and elbows out to about 90 degrees from your body. This position will place more stress on the deltoids and pecs. To get into this position place your hands a little wider than shoulder width. Rotate your elbows out to the side before descending. Sometimes it's easier to rotate the fingers slightly in towards your head although I have seen people do these pushups with fingers pointing out away from the body as well. This position can place a lot of stress on the pectorals so be careful not to overdo it and injure yourself.

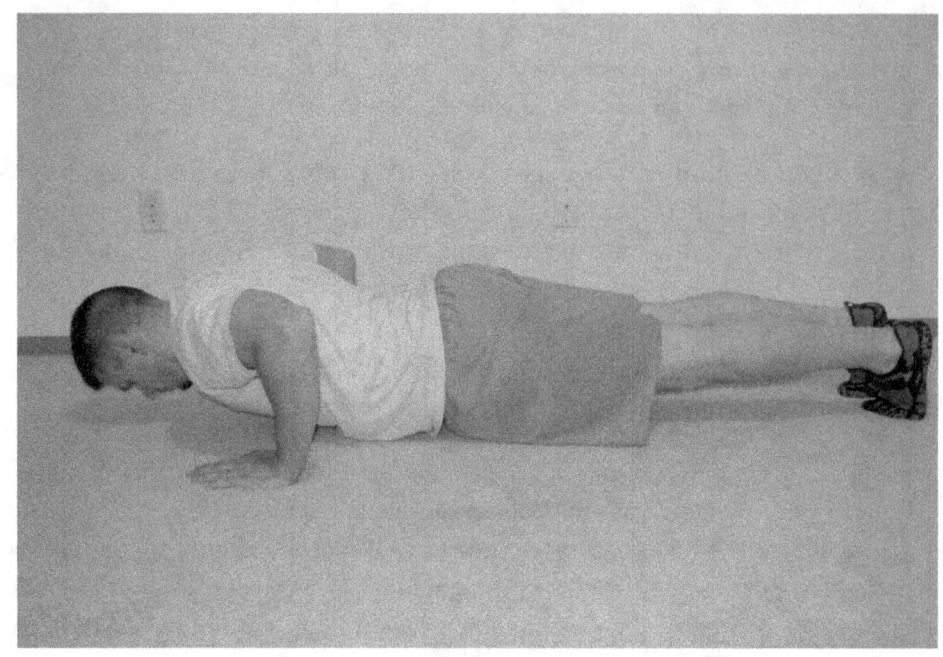

Position 1. Elbows at 45 degrees from the torso

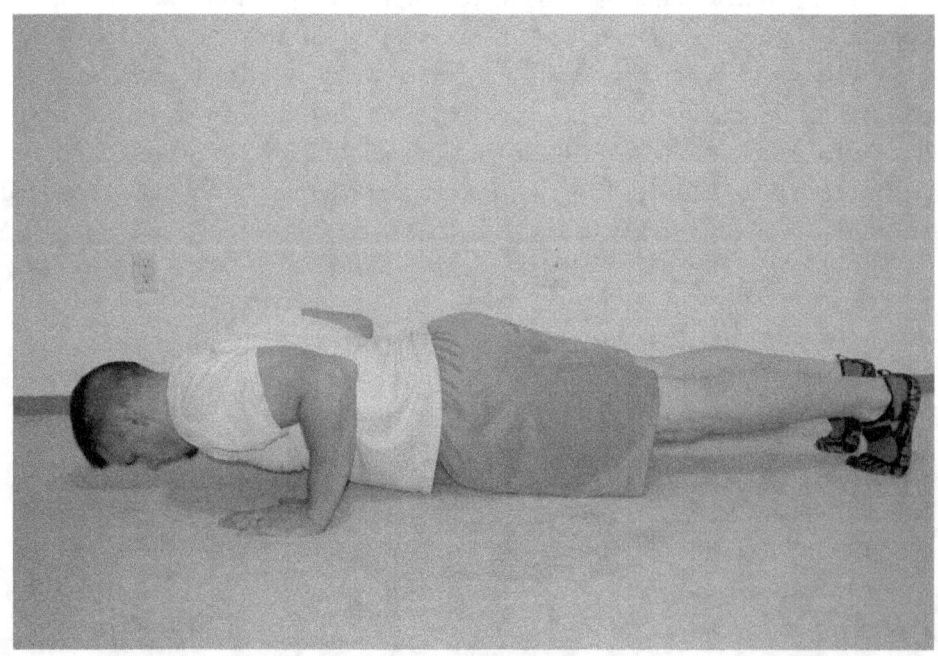

Position 2. Elbows in against the torso

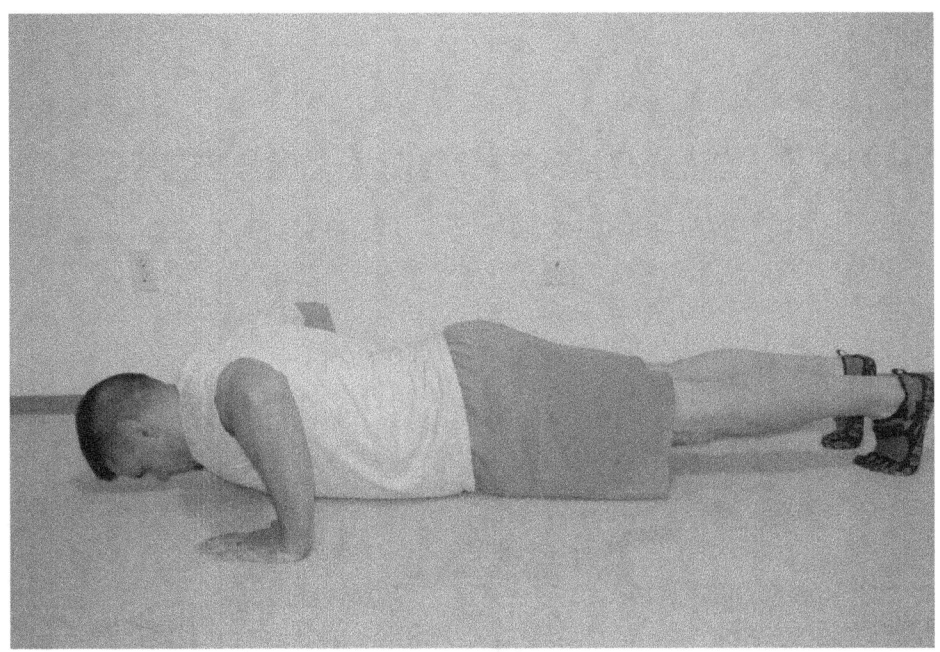
Position 3. Elbows out 90 degrees from the torso

Appendix C: Supplemental Exercises

List of Figures

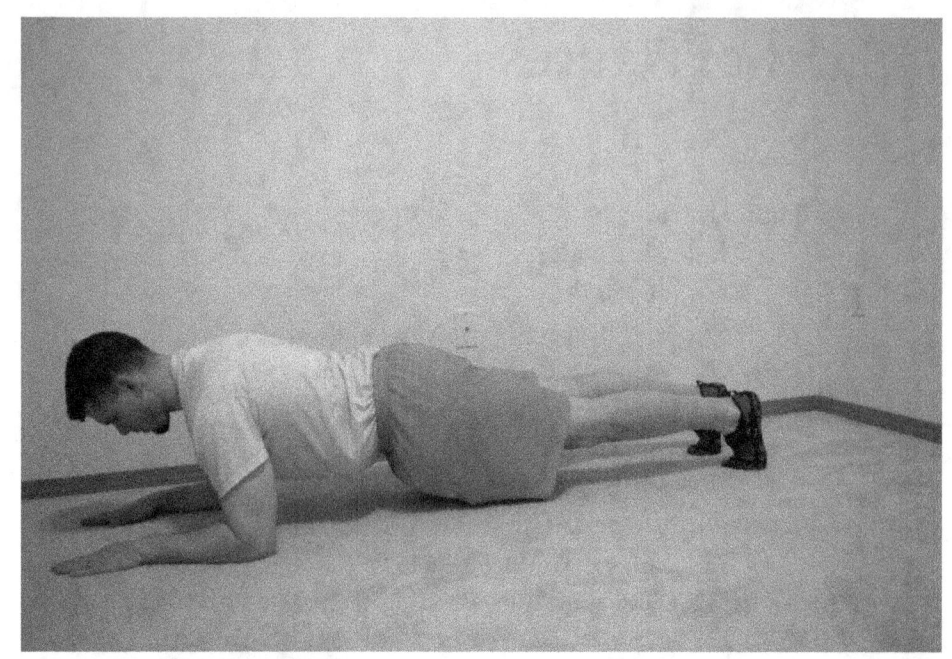

C1. Basic Plank

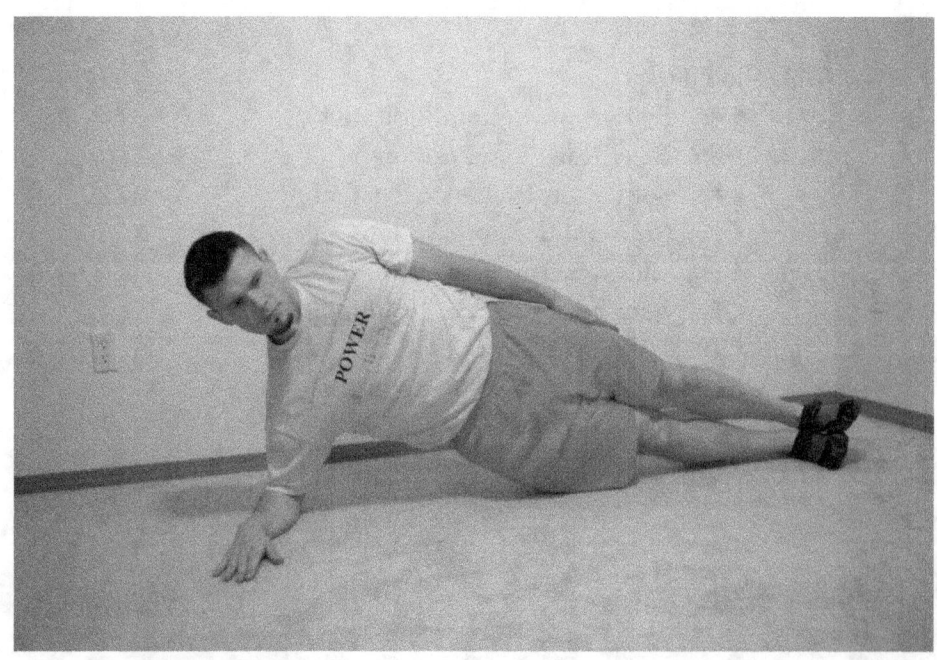

C2. Side Plank

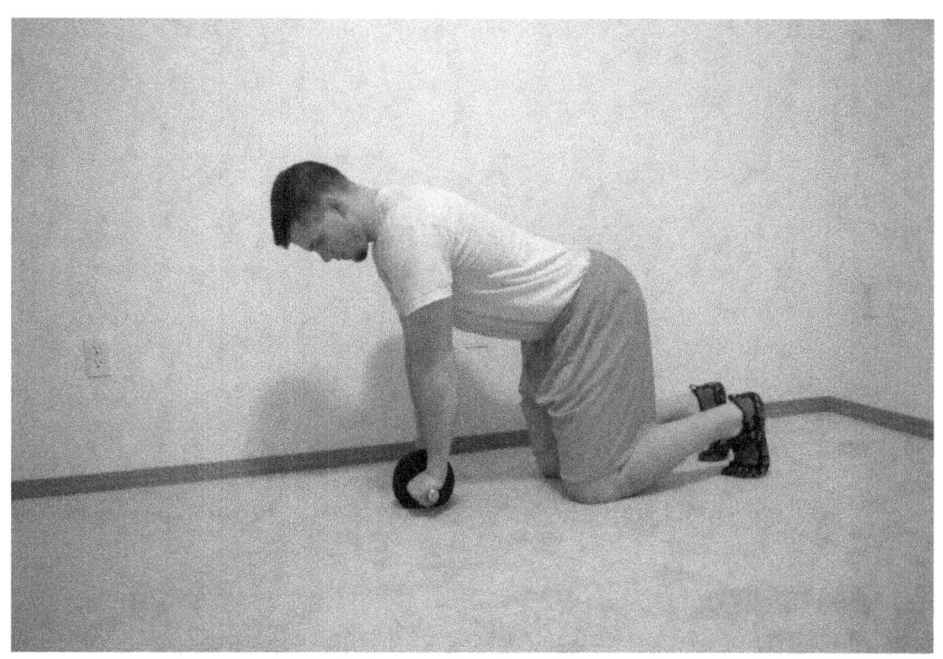

C3a. Ab-wheel Roll-out, Top Position

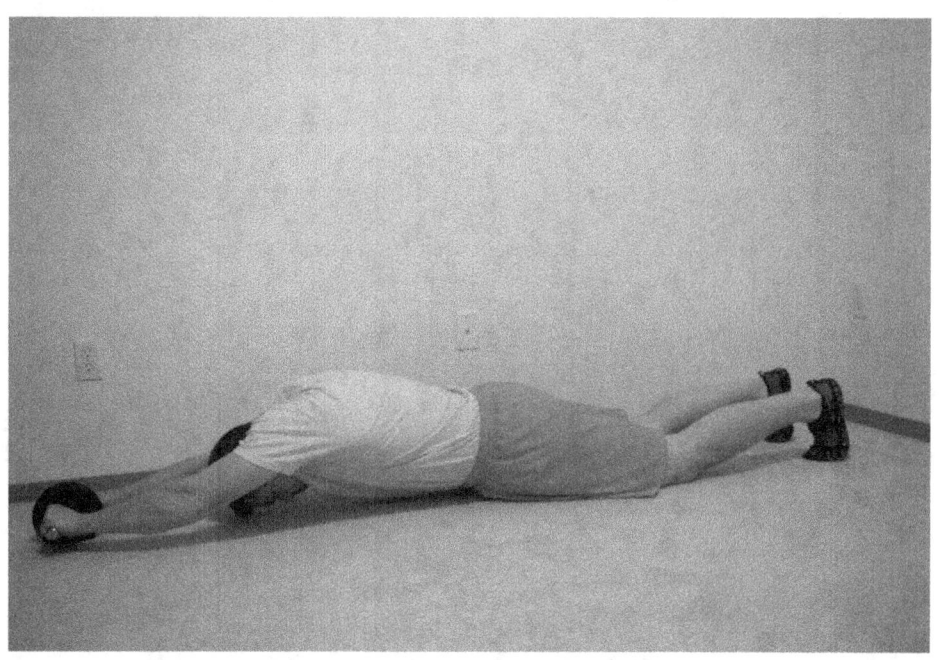

C3b. Ab-wheel Roll-out, Bottom Position

43

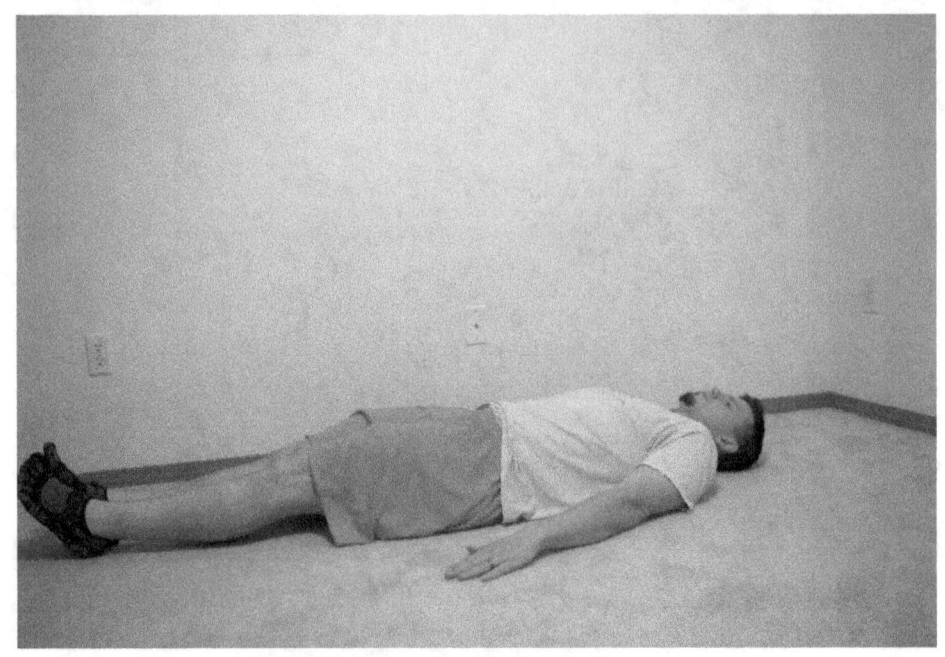

C4a. Leg Raises, Bottom Position

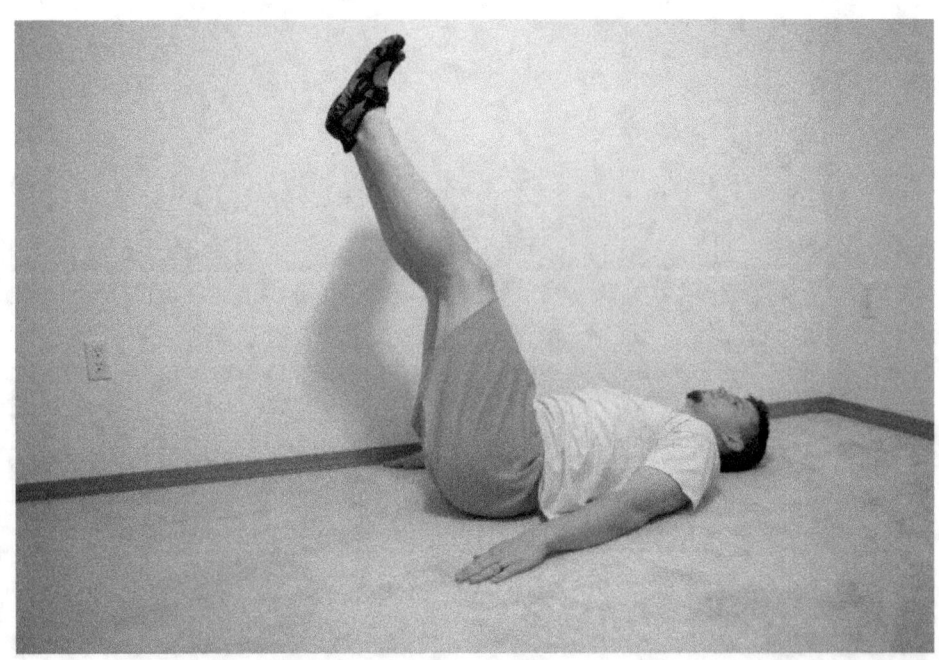

C4b. Leg Raises, Top Position

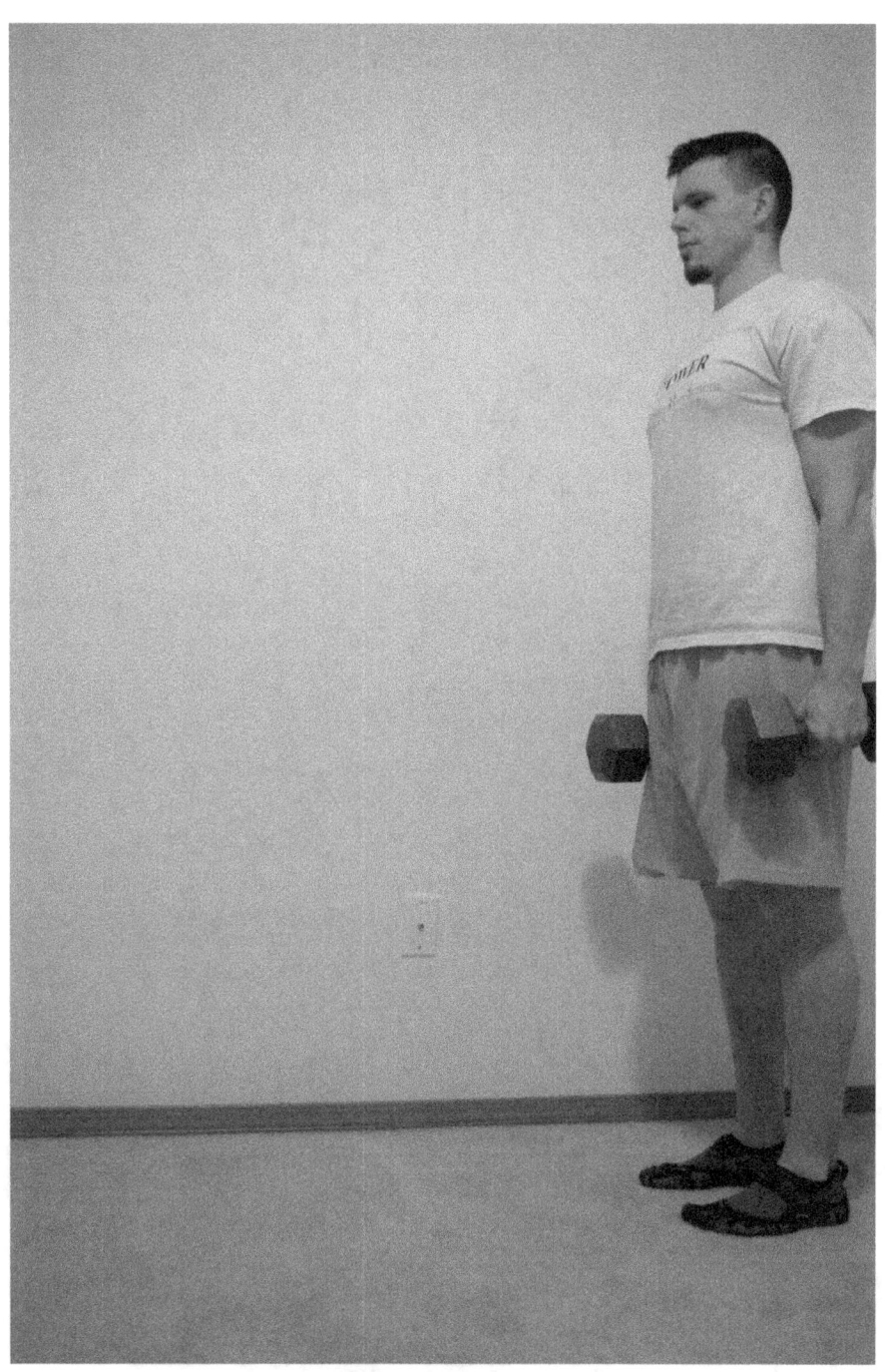

C5a. Lunges, Top Position

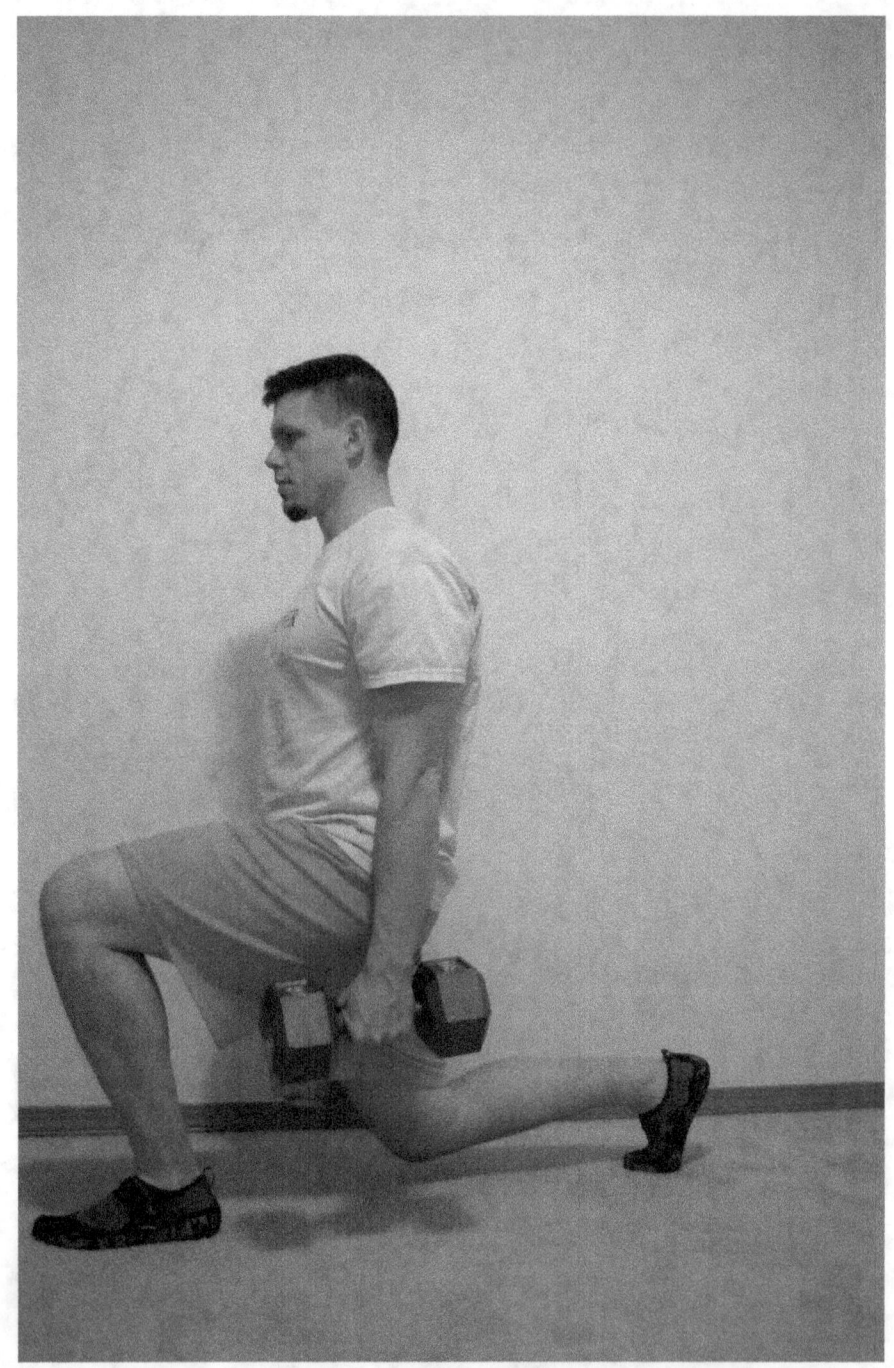

C5b. Lunges, Bottom Position/Isometric Position

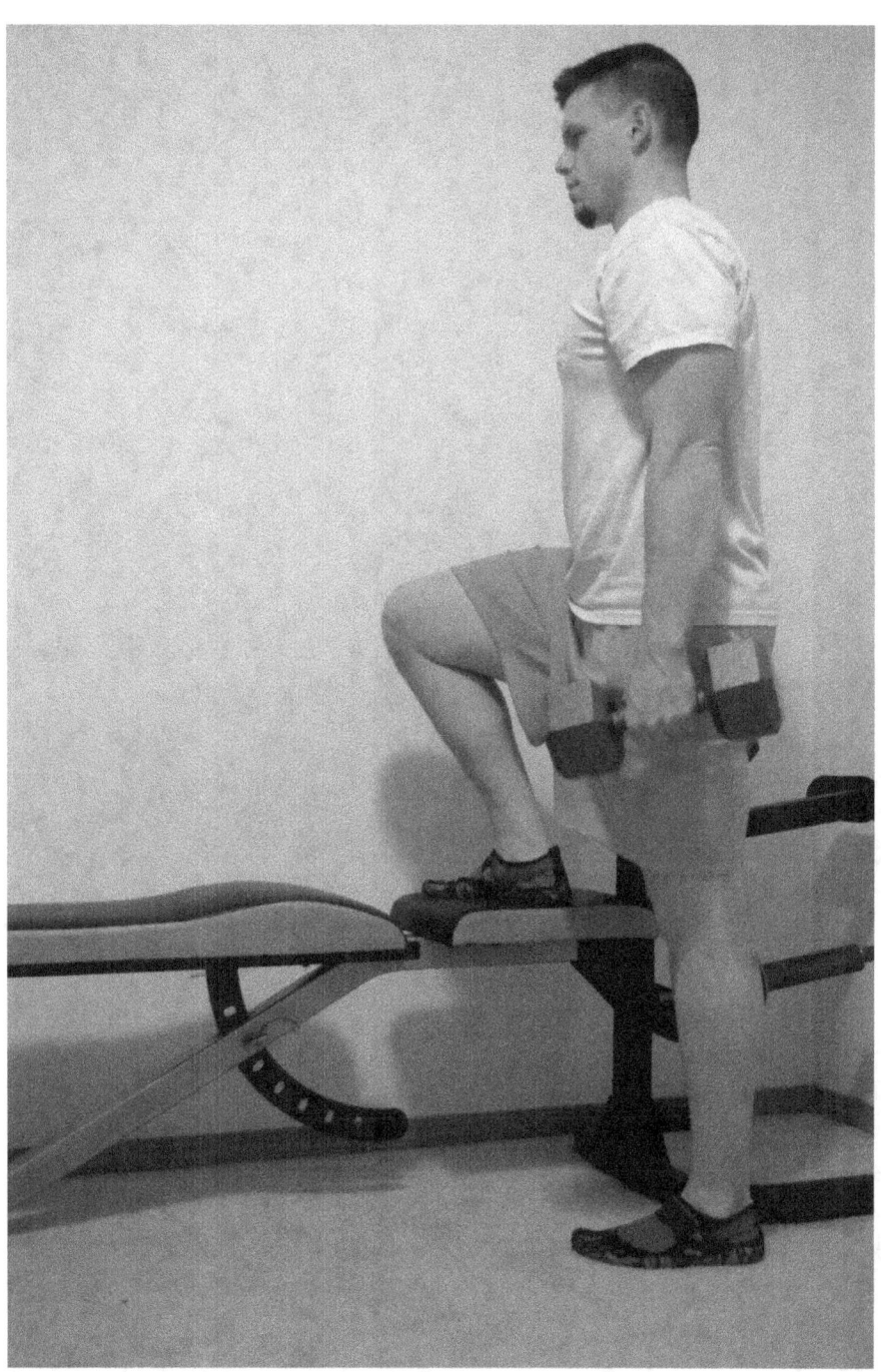

C6a. Step-ups, Bottom Position

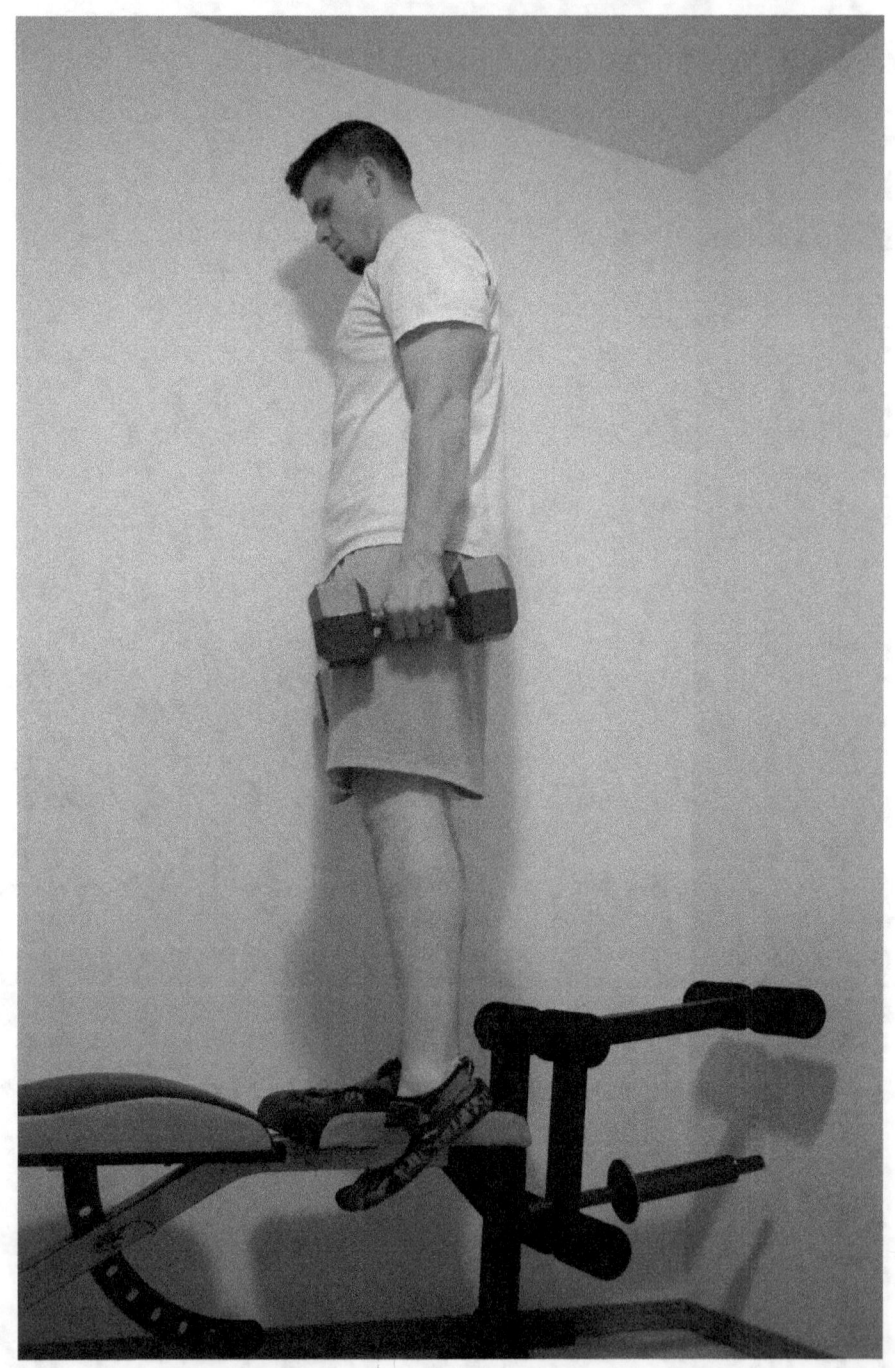

C6b. Step-ups, Top Position

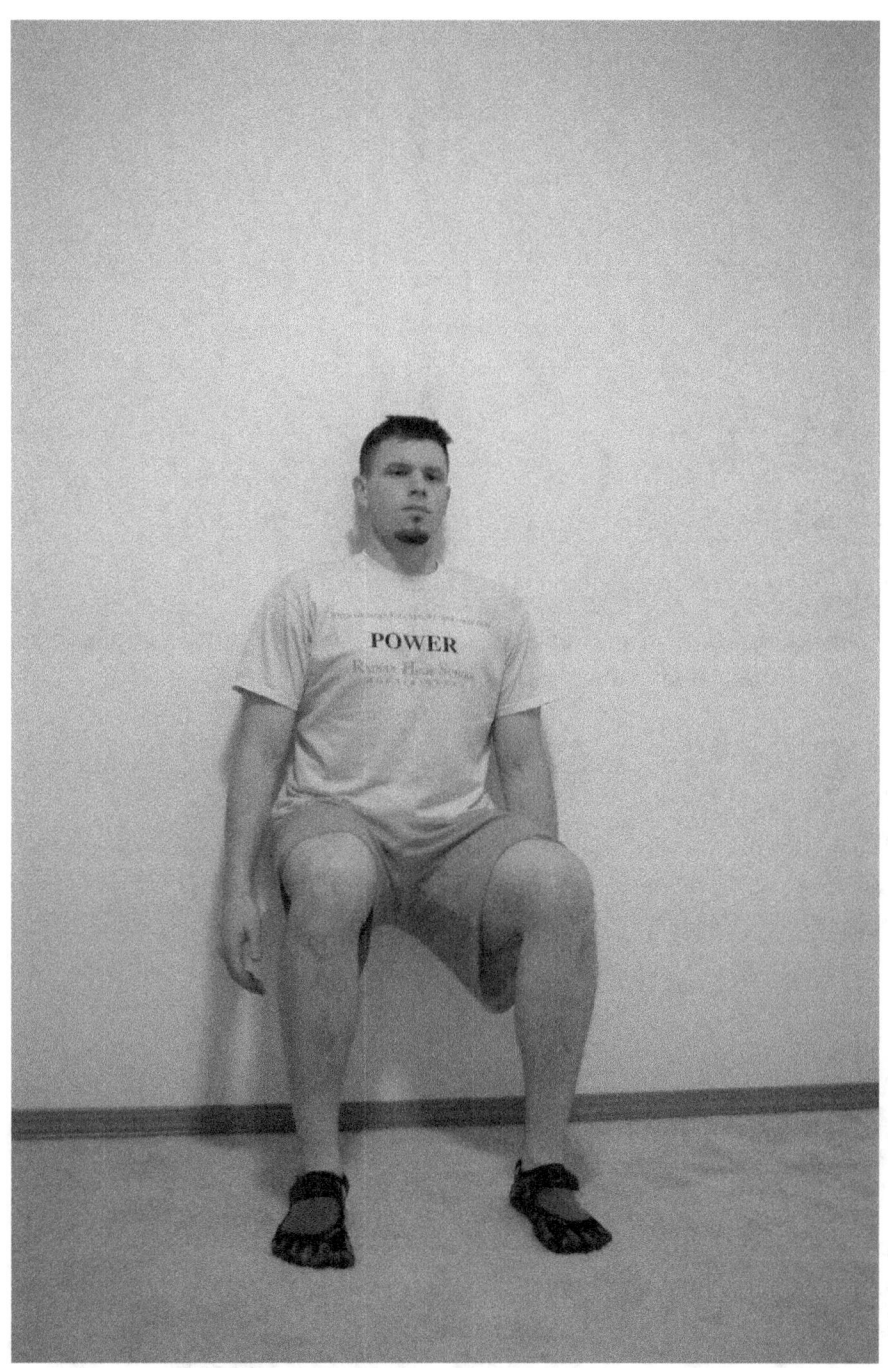

C7. Isometric Wall Sit

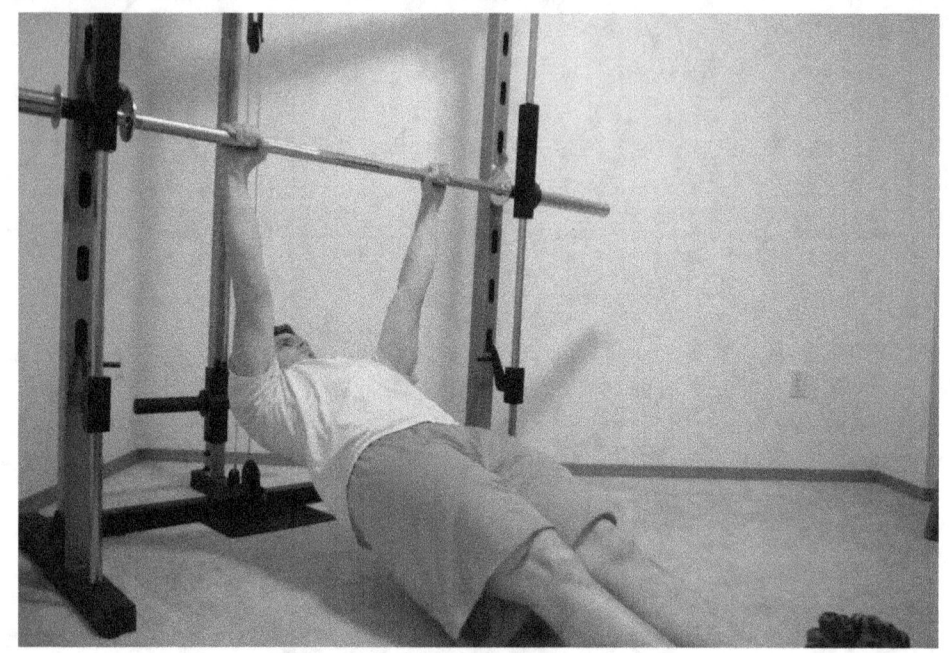

C8a. Body Row, Bottom Position

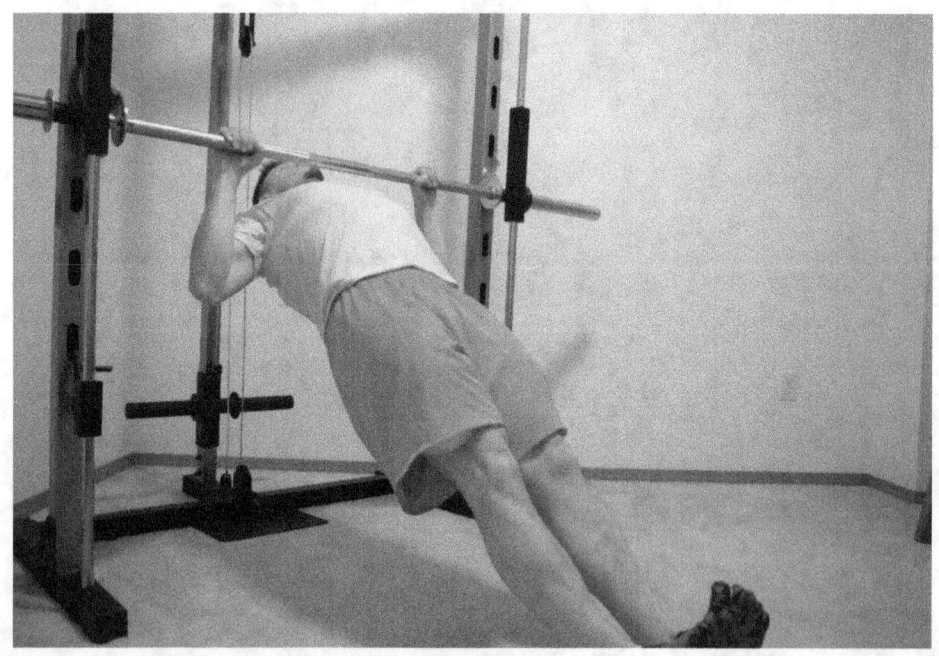

C8b. Body Row, Top Position

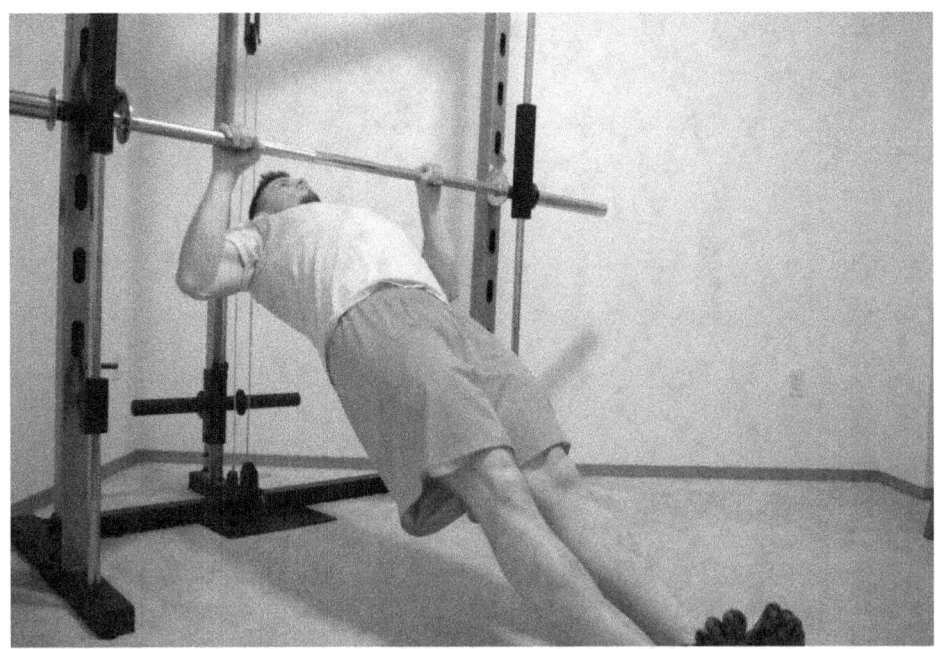

C8c. Body Row, Isometric Position

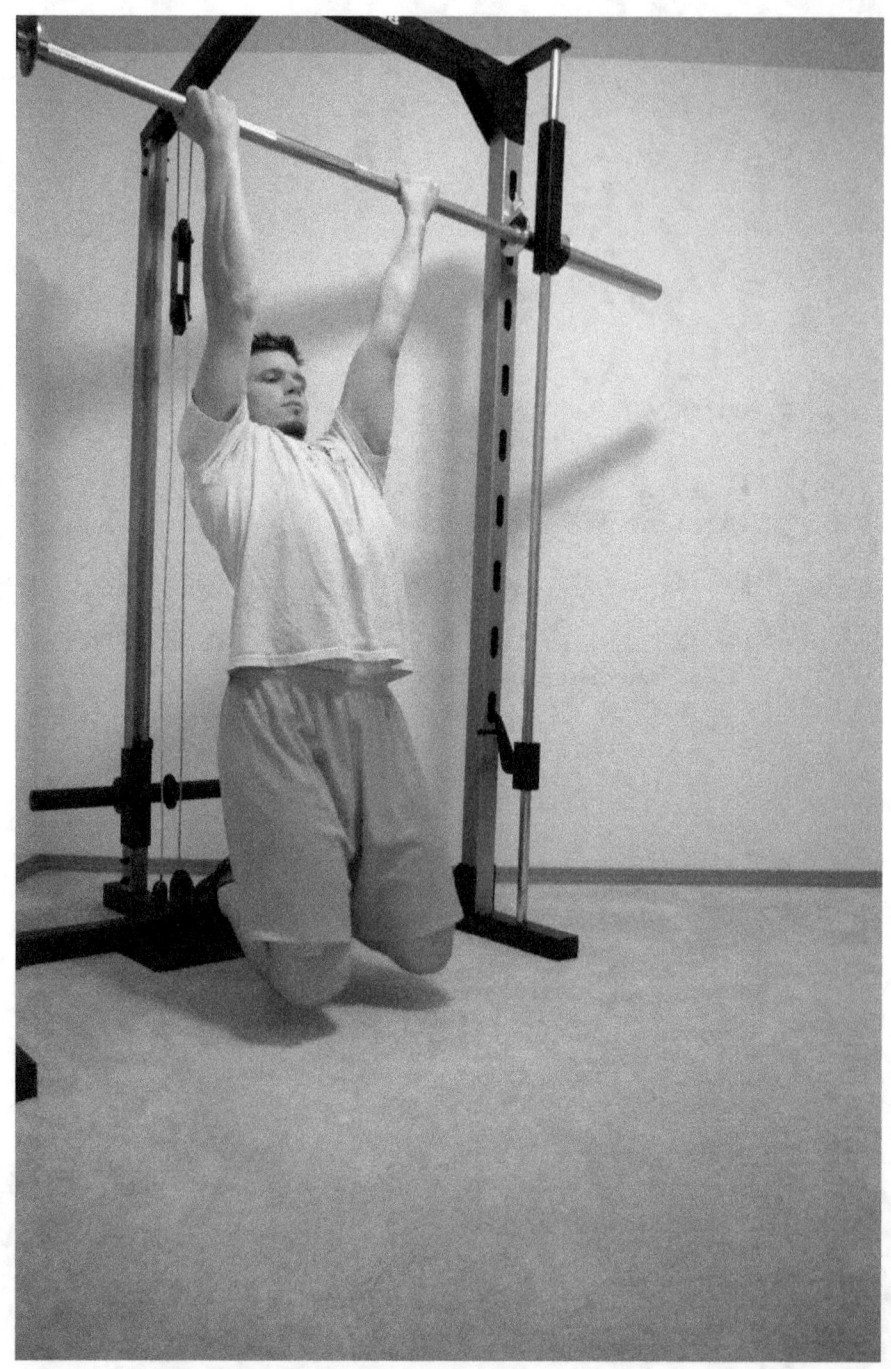

C9a. Chin-up, Bottom Position

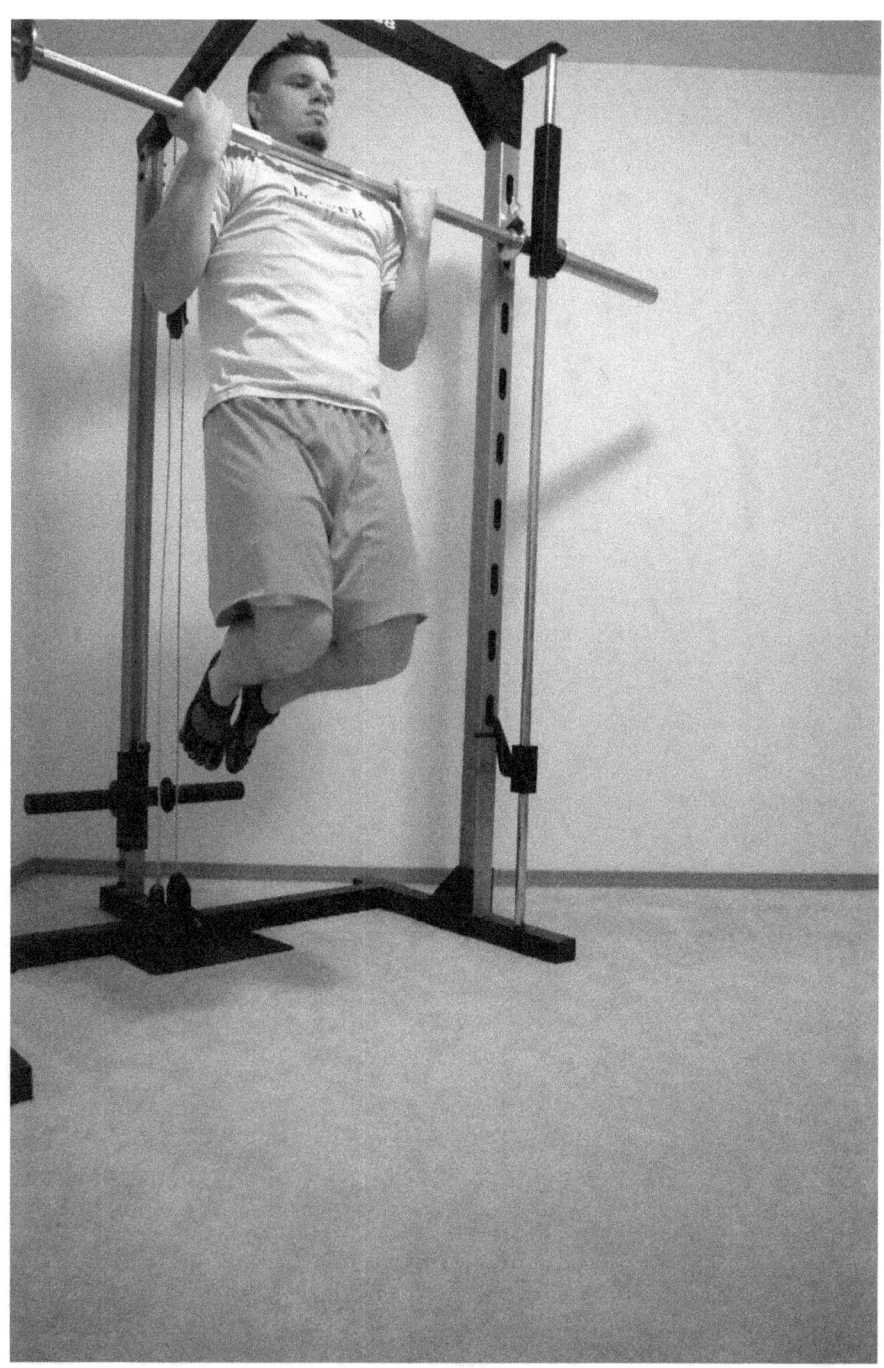

C9b. Chin-up, Top Position

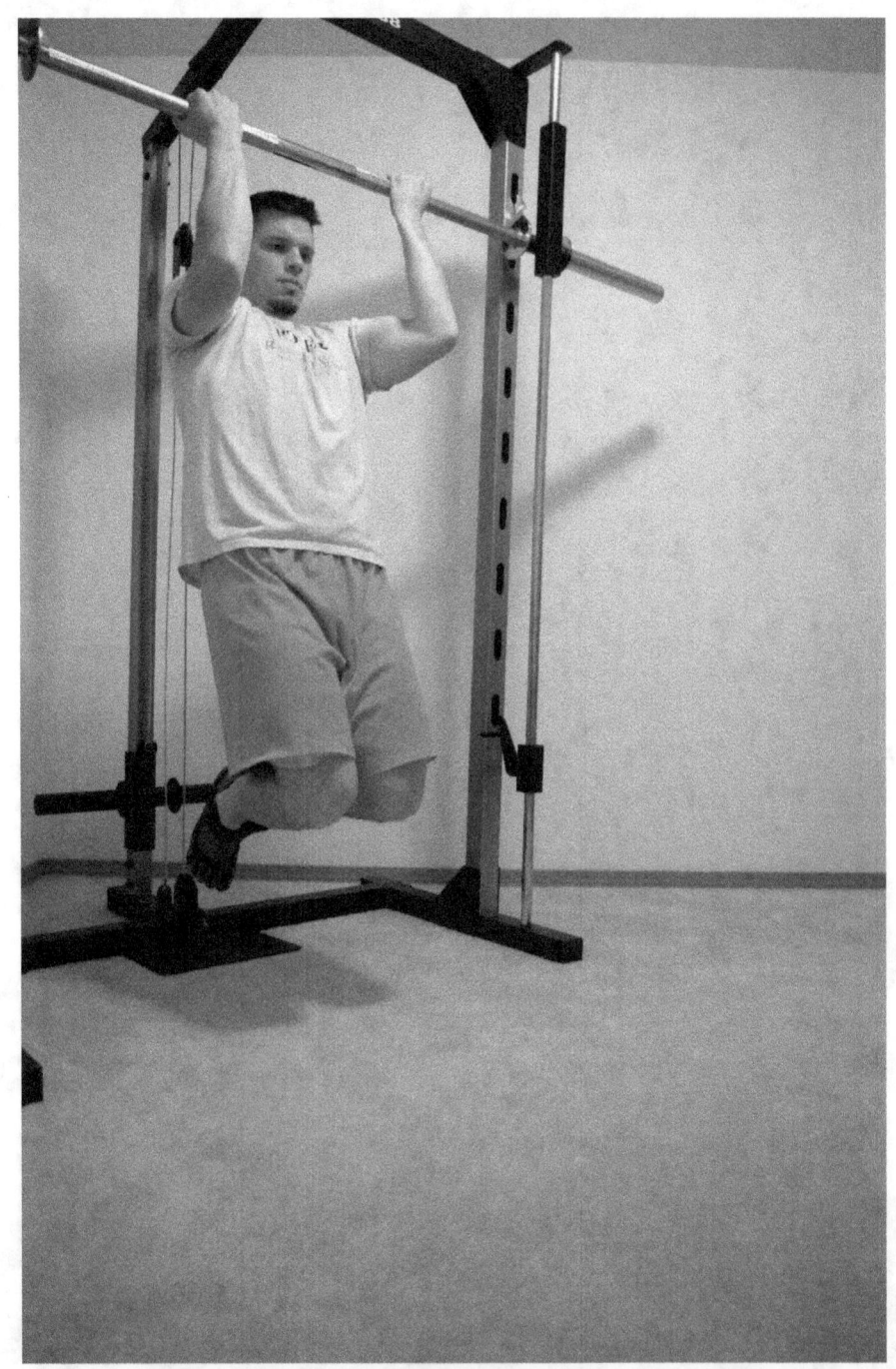

C9c. Chin-up, Isometric Position

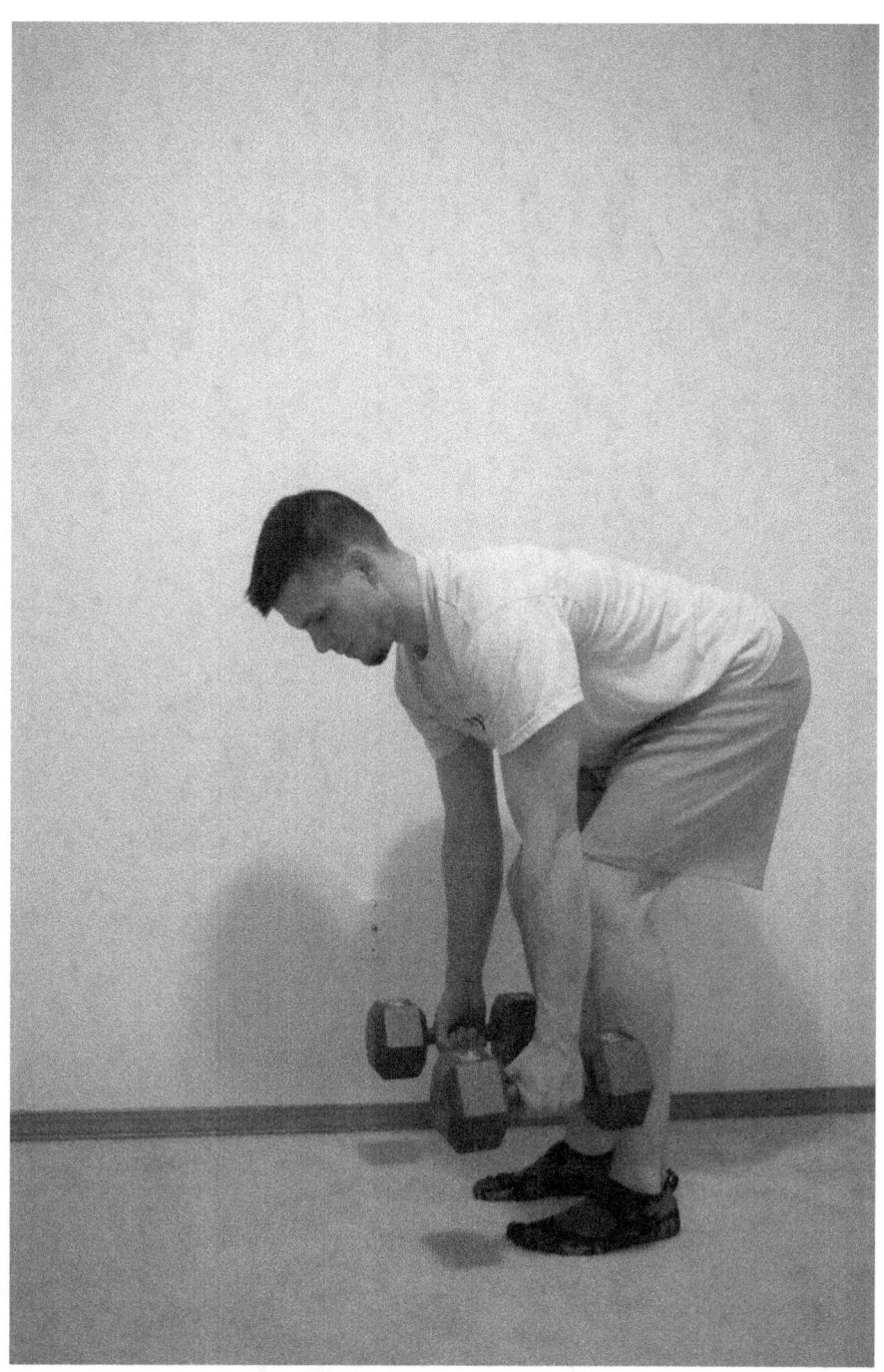

C10a. Dumbbell Rows, Bottom Position

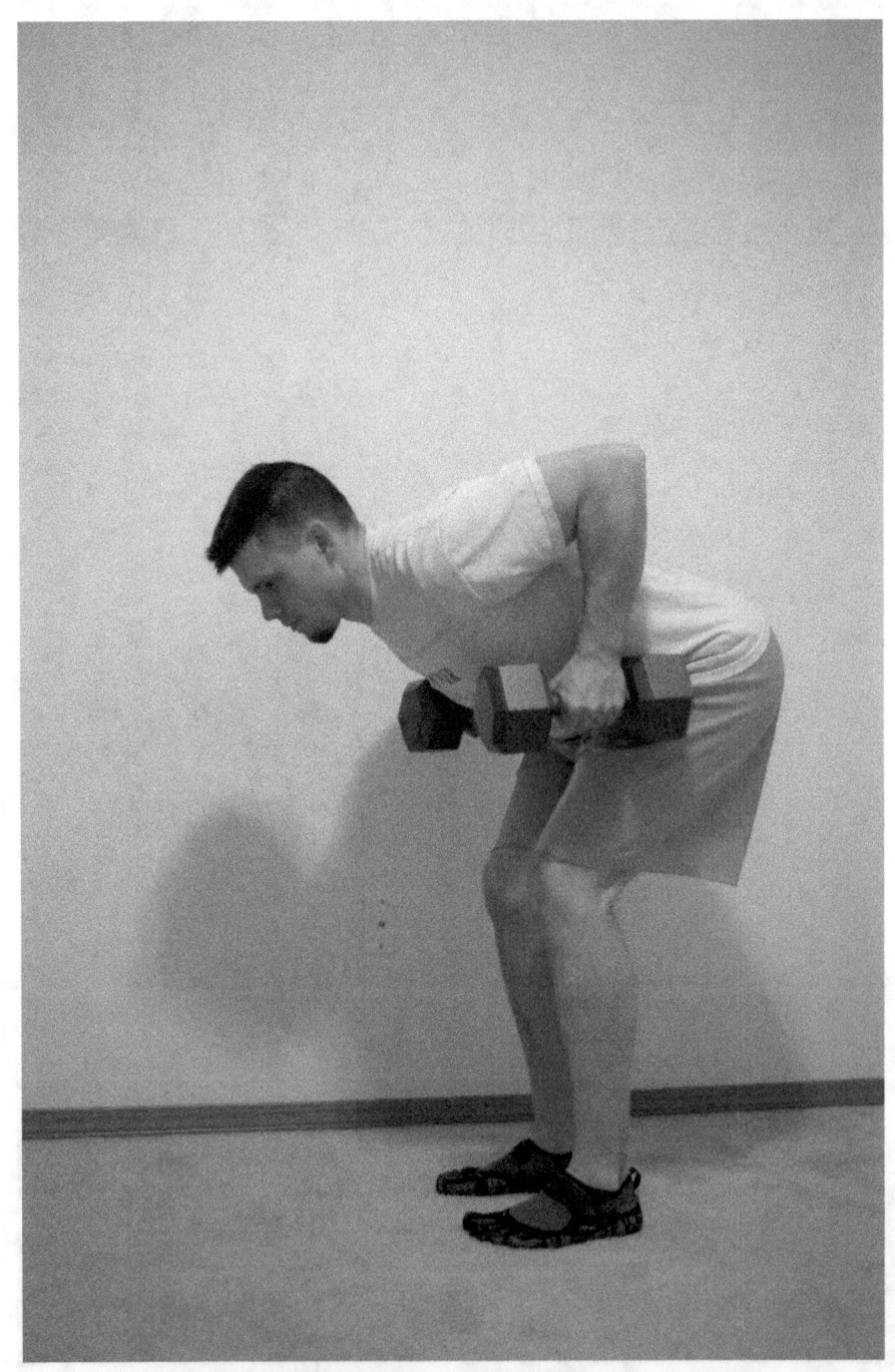

C10b. Dumbbell Rows, Top Position

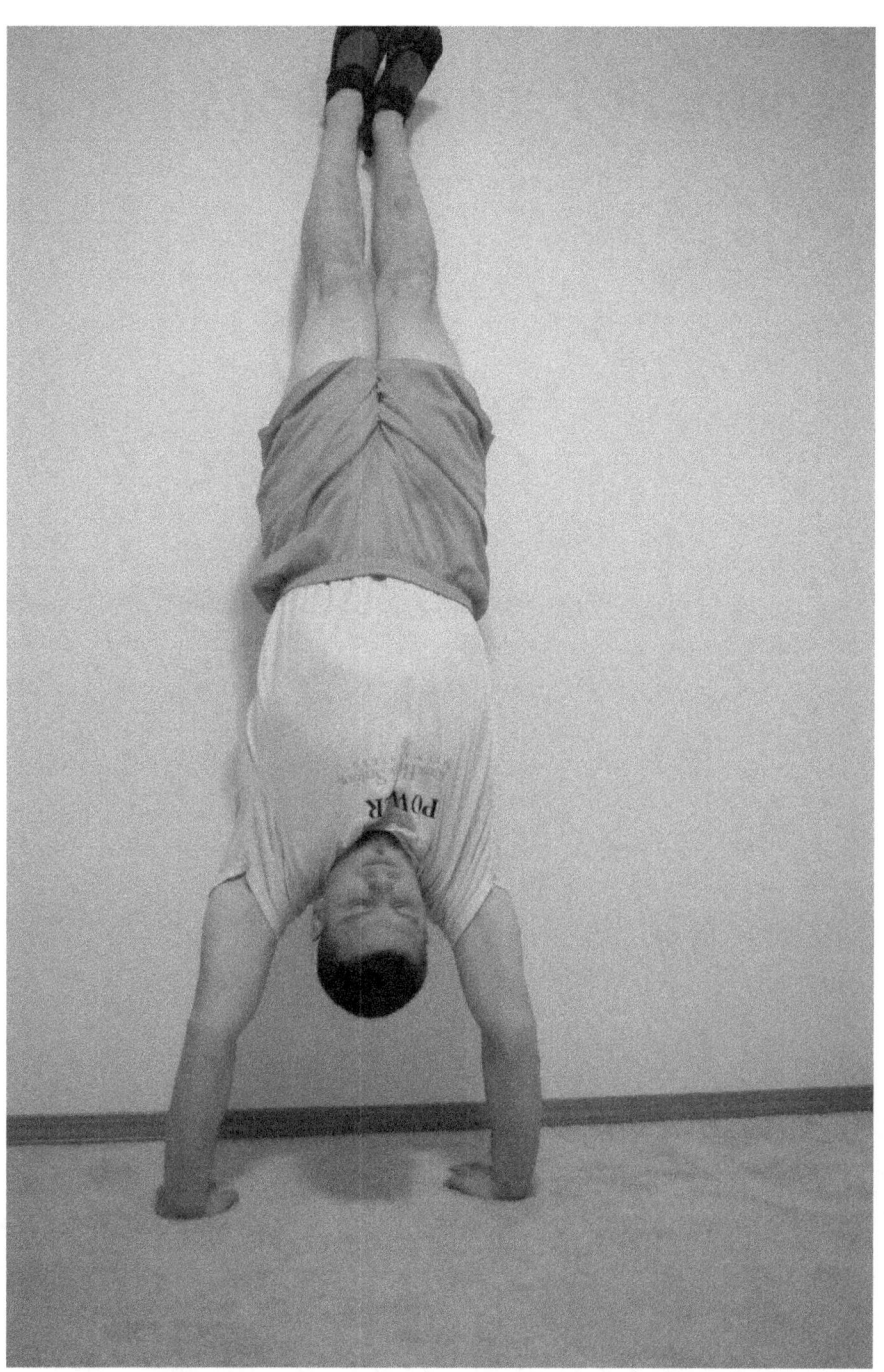

C11. Isometric Wall Handstands

Appendix D: Progress Logs

Week 1:

Day 1	Day 2	Day 3	Day 4	Day 5	Day 6	Day 7
Pushups Goal/Actual	Lunge Type: Time/Reps:	Pushups Goal/Actual	Handstands Time:	Lunge Type: Time/Reps:	Pushups Max	
1. /	1: :	1. /	1:	1: :	1:	
2. /	2: :	2. /	2:	2: :	2:	
3. /	3: :	3. /		3: :		
	4: :			4: :		
Abs Exercise: Time/Reps:	Rows/Pullups Exercise: Time/Reps:	Abs Exercise: Time/Reps:	Wallsits Time:	Rows/Pullups Exercise: Time/Reps:	Abs Exercise: Time/Reps:	
1: :	1: :	1: :	1:	1: :	1: :	
2: :	2: :	2: :		2: :		
3: :	3: :	3: :		3: :		

Week 2:

Day 1	Day 2	Day 3	Day 4	Day 5	Day 6	Day 7
Pushups Goal/Actual	Lunge Type: Time/Reps:	Pushups Goal/Actual	Handstands Time:	Lunge Type: Time/Reps:	Pushups Max	
1. /	1: :	1. /	1:	1: :	1:	
2. /	2: :	2. /	2:	2: :	2:	
3. /	3: :	3. /		3: :		
	4: :			4: :		
Abs Exercise: Time/Reps:	Rows/Pullups Exercise: Time/Reps:	Abs Exercise: Time/Reps:	Wallsits Time:	Rows/Pullups Exercise: Time/Reps:	Abs Exercise: Time/Reps:	
1: :	1: :	1: :	1:	1: :	1: :	
2: :	2: :	2: :		2: :		
3: :	3: :	3: :		3: :		

Week 3:

Day 1	Day 2	Day 3	Day 4	Day 5	Day 6	Day 7
Pushups Goal/Actual	Lunge Type: Time/Reps:	Pushups Goal/Actual	Handstands Time:	Lunge Type: Time/Reps:	Pushups Max	
1. /	1: :	1. /	1:	1: :	1:	
2. /	2: :	2. /	2:	2: :	2:	
3. /	3: :	3. /		3: :		
	4: :			4: :		
Abs Exercise: Time/Reps:	Rows/Pullups Exercise: Time/Reps:	Abs Exercise: Time/Reps:	Wallsits Time:	Rows/Pullups Exercise: Time/Reps:	Abs Exercise: Time/Reps:	
1: :	1: :	1: :	1:	1: :	1: :	
2: :	2: :	2: :		2: :		
3: :	3: :	3: :		3: :		

Week 4:

Day 1	Day 2	Day 3	Day 4	Day 5	Day 6	Day 7
Pushups Goal/Actual	Lunge Type: Time/Reps:	Pushups Goal/Actual	Handstands Time:	Lunge Type: Time/Reps:	Pushups Max	
1. /	1: :	1. /	1:	1: :	1:	
2. /	2: :	2. /	2:	2: :	2:	
3. /	3: :	3. /		3: :		
	4: :			4: :		
Abs Exercise: Time/Reps:	Rows/Pullups Exercise: Time/Reps:	Abs Exercise: Time/Reps:	Wallsits Time:	Rows/Pullups Exercise: Time/Reps:	Abs Exercise: Time/Reps:	
1: :	1: :	1: :	1:	1: :	1: :	
2: :	2: :	2: :		2: :		
3: :	3: :	3: :		3: :		

Week 5:

Day 1	Day 2	Day 3	Day 4	Day 5	Day 6	Day 7
Pushups Goal/Actual	Lunge Type: Time/Reps:	Pushups Goal/Actual	Handstands Time:	Lunge Type: Time/Reps:	Pushups Max	
1. /	1: :	1. /	1:	1: :	1:	
2. /	2: :	2. /	2:	2: :	2:	
3. /	3: :	3. /		3: :		
	4: :			4: :		
Abs Exercise: Time/Reps:	Rows/Pullups Exercise: Time/Reps:	Abs Exercise: Time/Reps:	Wallsits Time:	Rows/Pullups Exercise: Time/Reps:	Abs Exercise: Time/Reps:	
1: :	1: :	1: :	1:	1: :	1: :	
2: :	2: :	2: :		2: :		
3: :	3: :	3: :		3: :		

Week 6:

Day 1	Day 2	Day 3	Day 4	Day 5	Day 6	Day 7
Pushups Goal/Actual	Lunge Type: Time/Reps:	Pushups Goal/Actual	Handstands Time:	Lunge Type: Time/Reps:	Pushups Max	
1. /	1: :	1. /	1:	1: :	1:	
2. /	2: :	2. /	2:	2: :	2:	
3. /	3: :	3. /		3: :		
	4: :			4: :		
Abs Exercise: Time/Reps:	Rows/Pullups Exercise: Time/Reps:	Abs Exercise: Time/Reps:	Wallsits Time:	Rows/Pullups Exercise: Time/Reps:	Abs Exercise: Time/Reps:	
1: :	1: :	1: :	1:	1: :	1: :	
2: :	2: :	2: :		2: :		
3: :	3: :	3: :		3: :		

Week 7:

Day 1	Day 2	Day 3	Day 4	Day 5	Day 6	Day 7
Pushups Goal/Actual	Lunge Type: Time/Reps:	Pushups Goal/Actual	Handstands Time:	Lunge Type: Time/Reps:	Pushups Max	
1. /	1: :	1. /	1:	1: :	1:	
2. /	2: :	2. /	2:	2: :	2:	
3. /	3: :	3. /		3: :		
	4: :			4: :		
Abs Exercise: Time/Reps:	Rows/Pullups Exercise: Time/Reps:	Abs Exercise: Time/Reps:	Wallsits Time:	Rows/Pullups Exercise: Time/Reps:	Abs Exercise: Time/Reps:	
1: :	1: :	1: :	1:	1: :	1: :	
2: :	2: :	2: :		2: :		
3: :	3: :	3: :		3: :		

Week 8:

Day 1	Day 2	Day 3	Day 4	Day 5	Day 6	Day 7
Pushups Goal/Actual	Lunge Type: Time/Reps:	Pushups Goal/Actual	Handstands Time:	Lunge Type: Time/Reps:	Pushups Max	
1. /	1: :	1. /	1:	1: :	1:	
2. /	2: :	2. /	2:	2: :	2:	
3. /	3: :	3. /		3: :		
	4: :			4: :		
Abs Exercise: Time/Reps:	Rows/Pullups Exercise: Time/Reps:	Abs Exercise: Time/Reps:	Wallsits Time:	Rows/Pullups Exercise: Time/Reps:	Abs Exercise: Time/Reps:	
1: :	1: :	1: :	1:	1: :	1: :	
2: :	2: :	2: :		2: :		
3: :	3: :	3: :		3: :		

Week 9:

Day 1	Day 2	Day 3	Day 4	Day 5	Day 6	Day 7
Pushups Goal/Actual	Lunge Type: Time/Reps:	Pushups Goal/Actual	Handstands Time:	Lunge Type: Time/Reps:	Pushups Max	
1. /	1: :	1. /	1:	1: :	1:	
2. /	2: :	2. /	2:	2: :	2:	
3. /	3: :	3. /		3: :		
	4: :			4: :		
Abs Exercise: Time/Reps:	Rows/Pullups Exercise: Time/Reps:	Abs Exercise: Time/Reps:	Wallsits Time:	Rows/Pullups Exercise: Time/Reps:	Abs Exercise: Time/Reps:	
1: :	1: :	1: :	1:	1: :	1: :	
2: :	2: :	2: :		2: :		
3: :	3: :	3: :		3: :		

Week 10:

Day 1	Day 2	Day 3	Day 4	Day 5	Day 6	Day 7
Pushups Goal/Actual	Lunge Type: Time/Reps:	Pushups Goal/Actual	Handstands Time:	Lunge Type: Time/Reps:	Pushups Max	
1. /	1: :	1. /	1:	1: :	1:	
2. /	2: :	2. /	2:	2: :	2:	
3. /	3: :	3. /		3: :		
	4: :			4: :		
Abs Exercise: Time/Reps:	Rows/Pullups Exercise: Time/Reps:	Abs Exercise: Time/Reps:	Wallsits Time:	Rows/Pullups Exercise: Time/Reps:	Abs Exercise: Time/Reps:	
1: :	1: :	1: :	1:	1: :	1: :	
2: :	2: :	2: :		2: :		
3: :	3: :	3: :		3: :		

Week 11:

Day 1	Day 2	Day 3	Day 4	Day 5	Day 6	Day 7
Pushups Goal/Actual	Lunge Type: Time/Reps:	Pushups Goal/Actual	Handstands Time:	Lunge Type: Time/Reps:	Pushups Max	
1. /	1: :	1. /	1:	1: :	1:	
2. /	2: :	2. /	2:	2: :	2:	
3. /	3: :	3. /		3: :		
	4: :			4: :		
Abs Exercise: Time/Reps:	Rows/Pullups Exercise: Time/Reps:	Abs Exercise: Time/Reps:	Wallsits Time:	Rows/Pullups Exercise: Time/Reps:	Abs Exercise: Time/Reps:	
1: :	1: :	1: :	1:	1: :	1: :	
2: :	2: :	2: :		2: :		
3: :	3: :	3: :		3: :		

Week 12:

Day 1	Day 2	Day 3	Day 4	Day 5	Day 6	Day 7
Pushups Goal/Actual	Lunge Type: Time/Reps:	Pushups Goal/Actual	Handstands Time:	Lunge Type: Time/Reps:	Pushups Max	
1. /	1: :	1. /	1:	1: :	1:	
2. /	2: :	2. /	2:	2: :	2:	
3. /	3: :	3. /		3: :		
	4: :			4: :		
Abs Exercise: Time/Reps:	Rows/Pullups Exercise: Time/Reps:	Abs Exercise: Time/Reps:	Wallsits Time:	Rows/Pullups Exercise: Time/Reps:	Abs Exercise: Time/Reps:	
1: :	1: :	1: :	1:	1: :	1: :	
2: :	2: :	2: :		2: :		
3: :	3: :	3: :		3: :		

www.ingramcontent.com/pod-product-compliance
Lightning Source LLC
Chambersburg PA
CBHW081850280526
45789CB00007B/2643